Clinical Genetics:
A Case-based Approach

Clinical Genetics:
A Case-based Approach

David T Bonthron
BA MRCP
Senior Lecturer in Human Genetics
Western General Hospital
Edinburgh
UK

David R FitzPatrick
MD MRCP
Consultant Clinical Geneticist
Western General Hospital
Edinburgh
UK

Mary E M Porteous
MSc MD MRCP
Consultant Clinical Geneticist
Western General Hospital
Edinburgh
UK

Alison H Trainer
BSc MSc MRCP
Specialist Registrar
The Duncan Guthrie Institute of Medical Genetics
Yorkhill NHS Trust
Glasgow
UK

WB Saunders Company Limited
London Philadelphia Toronto Sydney Tokyo

W.B. Saunders Company Ltd 24–28 Oval Road
London NW1 7DX

The Curtis Center
Independence Square West
Philadelphia, PA 19106-3399, USA

Harcourt Brace & Company
55 Horner Avenue
Toronto, Ontario M8Z 4X6, Canada

Harcourt Brace & Company, Australia
30–52 Smidmore Street
Marrickville, NSW 2204, Australia

Harcourt Brace & Company, Japan
Ichibancho Central Building, 22-1 Ichibancho
Chiyoda-ku, Tokyo 102, Japan

A catalogue record for this book is available from the British Library

ISBN 0-7020-2351-5

Typeset by Wyvern 21 Ltd, Bristol
Printed in Great Britain by The Bath Press, Bath

Contents

Preface

Research in the field of genetics has progressed so rapidly in recent years that it has become difficult for students and medical practitioners alike to know just where to begin. The present volume is intended to fill the need for a coherent and assessible introduction to the subject, and to outline basic clinical procedures. In doing so, it takes as its starting point not the DNA molecule or the chromosome, but the interests and anxieties of the presenting patient.

Each chapter anticipates and answers common questions, suggesting diagnostic procedures and therapies, with salient features highlighted in the accompanying boxes. The range of contributions reflects the authors' skill and experience in the hope of stimulating the reader's enthusiasm for this developing subject.

David T Bonthron
David R FitzPatrick
Mary E M Porteous
Alison H Trainer

Acknowledgements

The authors wish to acknowledge and thank the following for their contributions:

Mrs Elizabeth Grace Figs 2.1, 2.4, 9.8 and 9.9

Dr Shelagh Boyle Fig. 2.9a

Dr Jon P Warner
Mr T Johnston } Fig 2.11a,b

Mrs Avril Morris Fig. 2.11c

Dr Lisa Strain Figs 4.4b, 6.10, 7.5b and 8.8c

Dr Allan Stevenson Fig. 5.3

Dr Robin Sellar Fig. 5.5

Dr Lena Macara Figs 6.1, 6.2a, 6.3 and 6.5

Dr Sarah Chambers Fig. 6.2c

Dr David Gilmore Fig. 6.4a

Dr Alan Howatson Fig. 6.6

Dr Nick Smith Fig. 6.7

Dr Kate Bushby Fig. 7.6

Dr Jon P Warner and Ms Lilias Barron Fig. 8.11

Ms Jan Johnson Fig. 9.3

Professor John Burn Figs 9.4 and 9.5

Mr Malcolm Dunlop Fig. 9.6

I

The Family History

LEARNING OBJECTIVES

After studying this chapter, the reader should understand:

- how to draw an accurate family tree
- how to identify likely inheritance patterns from family trees

- the principles of genetic counselling

INTRODUCTION

A good understanding of the principles of inheritance is becoming increasingly important in all medical disciplines as more genetic factors underlying diseases are identified. As well as diseases caused by single-gene defects, common diseases such as dementia, ischaemic heart disease and type II diabetes mellitus also have established genetic predisposing factors.

The family history is an important part of a medical history and may point to a specific genetic diagnosis, thus avoiding unpleasant and expensive investigations. In addition a good family history may also identify disease susceptibilities that can be modified by treatment, for instance dietary modification and cholesterol lowering drug therapy in early coronary heart disease due to hypercholesterolaemia.

Genetic counselling is the process whereby an individual is informed of his/her risk of developing a disorder, the risk of passing it on to offspring and the options regarding testing and treatment. The basis for an initial genetic counselling appointment is the family tree. Whilst most specialists are concerned with diagnosing and treating individual patients, clinical geneticists have a responsibility both to the patient and the wider family. An accurate family tree is vital for the identification of individuals possibly at risk of developing a disorder or having children affected by the disorder.

HOW TO DRAW AN ACCURATE FAMILY TREE

Taking a family history

Before embarking on any genetic counselling, it is vital that accurate information is collected about as many family members as possible. This information is recorded in the form of a family tree. Information is usually collected from the consultand (the individual requesting genetic counselling). Frequently other members of the family have to be asked to provide additional detail, and it is helpful to warn people about the information that will be required before drawing up the family tree.

Drawing up the family tree together with the consultand serves four main purposes:

- establishment of a rapport between consultand and counsellor
- demonstration of mode of inheritance of the particular disease in the family

- provision of information on family relationships with identification of other individuals who may be at risk
- identification of the consultand's concerns and perceptions of the disease

It is important to find out the basis for the diagnosis in any identified affected individuals and this may involve contacting other professionals involved in their care. Confidentiality is essential and information must not be given to other family members without the patient's consent.

Remember, accurate counselling depends on accurate information and drawing a family tree is the first step towards collecting that information.

The following information should be provided for as many relatives as possible:

- full name (including maiden name)
- date of birth
- date and cause of death
- number of children and miscarriages
- any specific medical diagnoses

Tips for drawing a good family tree

- start in the middle of the page
- try to get information on three generations
- ask about consanguinity (see text)
- remember to include stillbirths and miscarriages

The standard convention for symbols (**Box 1.1**) should be used so that family trees can be understood by everyone involved in the family's care. The convention is to draw the male partner on the left and to list children from left to right from oldest to youngest. Although the consultand may not volunteer information about miscarriages, this is important information and should be asked for specifically.

An enquiry should be made as to consanguinity, that is if a couple are blood relatives. Blood relatives share a proportion of the same genes and offspring of consanguineous parents will have a higher risk of inheriting the same faulty gene from each parent. For instance, first cousins have 1 in 8 of their genes in common. **Box 1.2** shows different patterns of relationship and percentage of genes shared.

Consanguinity is an important consideration in autosomal recessive conditions which are discussed more fully later in the chapter.

HOW TO IDENTIFY LIKELY INHERITANCE PATTERNS FROM FAMILY TREES

Having drawn up the family tree the counsellor should determine whether the pattern of disease that is shown is likely to be 'genetic'. In this context 'genetic' means that a disease is due to a fault in one or both copies of a gene or is due to a chromosomal abnormality (see Chapter 2). Some diseases are multifactorial which means that they are due to an interaction between one or more pairs of genes and an environmental factor. Such conditions include spina bifida and epilepsy.

Single gene disorders

Each individual has nearly 100 000 pairs of genes or 'units of inheritance' which are bundled into 23 pairs of chromosomes comprising 22 pairs, termed autosomes and numbered 1 to 22 by decreasing size, and one pair of sex chromosomes (XX female, XY male). One member of each pair will have been inherited from the mother and one from the father and one or other of these is passed on to each of the children.

Single gene disorders are caused by a mutation or fault in one or both members of a pair of genes. They can be dominant (one normal copy and one faulty copy leads to the disease) or recessive (both copies must be faulty to produce symptoms and signs of the disease). Diseases caused by gene faults on the X chromosome are called sex-linked disorders. If a gene fault occurs in an X-linked gene, males will develop the disease as they have only one copy of the gene whilst females are usually protected by a second, normal copy. Specific features of each type of single gene disorder are given below.

Autosomal dominant disorders

The characteristic features of an autosomal dominant disease which can be detected in the family tree are:

BOX 1.1 STANDARD SYMBOLS USED IN DRAWING A FAMILY TREE

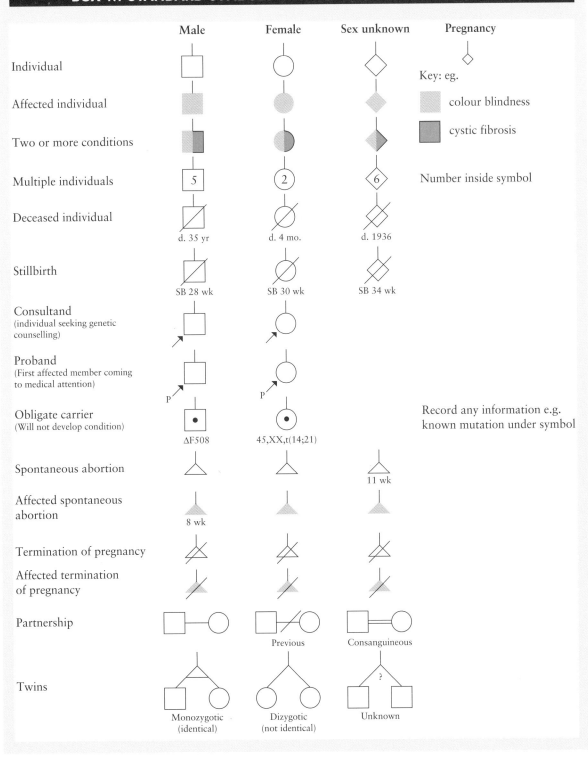

| | Male | Female | Sex unknown | Pregnancy |

Individual

Affected individual

Key: eg.
 colour blindness
 cystic fibrosis

Two or more conditions

Multiple individuals — 5, 2, 6 — Number inside symbol

Deceased individual — d. 35 yr, d. 4 mo., d. 1936

Stillbirth — SB 28 wk, SB 30 wk, SB 34 wk

Consultand
(individual seeking genetic counselling)

Proband
(First affected member coming to medical attention) — P, P

Obligate carrier
(Will not develop condition) — ΔF508, 45,XX,t(14;21)

Record any information e.g. known mutation under symbol

Spontaneous abortion — 11 wk

Affected spontaneous abortion — 8 wk

Termination of pregnancy

Affected termination of pregnancy

Partnership — Previous, Consanguineous

Twins — Monozygotic (identical), Dizygotic (not identical), ? Unknown

BOX 1.2 PERCENTAGE OF GENES SHARED BY BLOOD RELATIVES IN A FAMILY

Relationship		Percentage of genes shared
First degree relatives		
	Monozygotic (identical) twins	100%
	Parent–child	50%
	Dizygotic (non identical) twins	50%
	Siblings	50%
Second degree relatives		
	Half siblings	25%
	Aunt (uncle) – nephew (niece)	25%
	Double first cousins	25%
Third degree relatives		
	First cousins	12.5%

- involvement of more than one generation
- transmission of the disease from father to son (male to male transmission) can occur
- males and females affected with equal frequency and severity

An individual with an autosomal dominant disorder has a 1 in 2 chance of passing it on to his/her children whether male or female (**Box 1.3**).

An example of a typical autosomal dominant family tree is shown in Fig. 1.1.

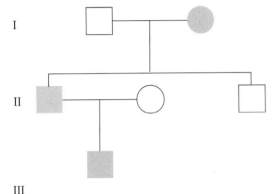

Fig. 1.1 A typical autosomal dominant family tree.

This family tree shows three generations of a family. The shaded symbols represent individuals who have symptoms and signs of a specific genetic disease. We can deduce that this disease has an autosomal dominant mode of inheritance as there are affected individuals in more than one generation and individual II-1 has passed it on to his son III-1.

Not all autosomal dominant family trees are as simple as the one described above. Consider the family tree shown in Fig. 1.2.

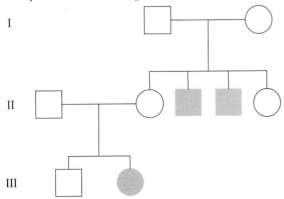

Fig. 1.2 Autosomal dominant family tree showing the presence of a non-penetrant gene carrier.

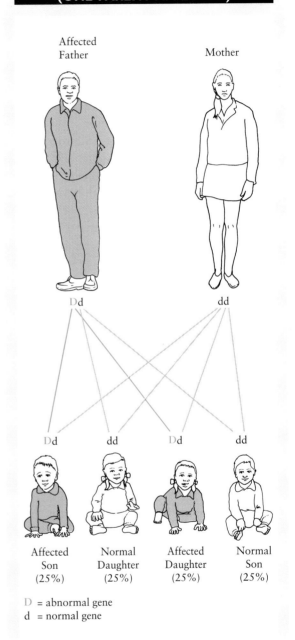

BOX 1.3 AUTOSOMAL DOMINANT INHERITANCE (ONE PARENT AFFECTED)

D = abnormal gene
d = normal gene

In this family tree the condition appears to have been passed on by an unaffected individual II-2. If all the shaded individuals have the same disease, then individual II-2 must carry the faulty gene but apparently shows no features of the disease.

This phenomenon can be explained in two ways, either II-2 has no clinical signs of the disease despite having the mutated gene, or she has a very mild form of the disease which may not have been diagnosed. When an individual carries a dominant mutation but shows no clinical signs of the disorder, s/he is called a non-penetrant gene carrier. Some disorders like achondroplasia, the commonest single-gene cause of disproportionate short stature, are known to be fully penetrant, i.e. all gene carriers manifest the condition.

Some autosomal dominant disorders have variable expressivity which means that affected individuals in the same family are affected to different degrees. For example, a mother with the autosomal dominant disease tuberous sclerosis (see Appendix II) may only have mild skin manifestations whilst her affected child has skin signs, severe seizures and learning difficulties. She may therefore be classed on the family tree as 'unaffected' if the subtle signs are not specifically looked for.

Autosomal recessive disorders

The typical features of an autosomal recessive family tree are:

- one or more affected children with unaffected parents
- usually only one generation involved
- males and females affected with equal frequency and severity
- a higher incidence of consanguinity

A typical autosomal recessive family tree is shown in Fig. 1.3.

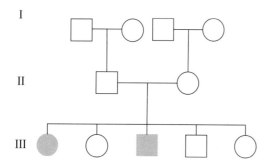

Fig. 1.3 A typical autosomal recessive family tree.

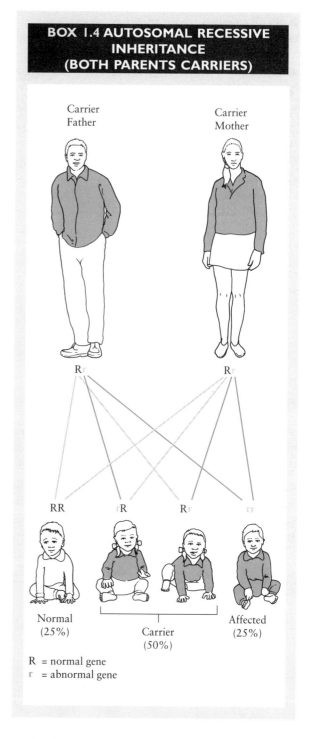

BOX 1.4 AUTOSOMAL RECESSIVE INHERITANCE (BOTH PARENTS CARRIERS)

Carrier Father   Carrier Mother

Rr   Rr

RR   rR   Rr   rr

Normal (25%)   Carrier (50%)   Affected (25%)

R = normal gene
r = abnormal gene

In this family tree two unaffected parents (II-1 and II-2) have two affected children, a girl and a boy (III-1 and III-3). This disease therefore affects males and females and is likely to have an autosomal recessive inheritance pattern (**Box 1.4**).

For the parents of a child with an autosomal recessive condition, the risk of having another affected child is 1 in 4. As both parents must be carriers for the condition, i.e. they each have one normal and one abnormal copy of the gene, the chance of them each passing on their abnormal gene simultaneously is therefore 1 in 4, with a 1 in 4 chance of the child inheriting both normal copies of the gene and a 2 in 4 (1 in 2) chance of inheriting one normal and one abnormal copy of the gene.

The unaffected siblings of an affected child have a 2 in 3 chance of being carriers of the condition as the fourth possiblity of being affected has been ruled out but the chances of their partner carrying the same gene fault is usually low so that the risk to their offspring is low. The risk is significantly increased if the siblings have children by a blood relative.

X-linked inheritance

As women have two X chromosomes, they have two copies of each X-linked gene. Men, with only one X, have only one copy. Therefore, if a woman has a mutation in an X-linked gene she should have a second, normal copy of the gene and therefore will be protected from the clinical or phenotypic effects of the mutation. Whilst this is usually true at a clinical level, women carriers of X-linked mutations may have subtle signs of the condition that causes severe disease in their brothers and sons. The underlying mechanism for this is called X-inactivation and will be discussed in more detail in Chapter 7. Because of this phenomenon, it is more accurate to describe diseases associated with mutations in genes on the X chromosome as X-linked rather than X-linked dominant or X-linked recessive (**Box 1.5**).

Features in the family tree that suggest X-linked inheritance are:

● usually only males affected
● more than one generation involved with the disease appearing to pass through normal females
● no male to male transmission

An example of an X-linked family tree is shown in Fig. 1.4.

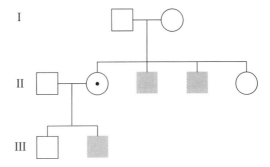

Fig. 1.4 An X-linked family tree.

The disease in this family seems to be transmitted by unaffected women, I-2 and II-2. As individual II-2 has two affected brothers (II-3 and II-4) as well as an affected son (III-2), the gene fault is likely to be on the X chromosome.

Individual II-2 is an obligate carrier of the X-linked disease running in the family because she has an affected son and two affected brothers. Her risk of having another affected boy in a future pregnancy is 1 in 4 (1 in 2 fetuses will be male and of these 1 in 2 will be affected). Her sister II-5 has a 1 in 2 risk of being a carrier based on the family tree alone, although in some X-linked diseases it is possible to perform other tests which will help to define her carrier risk more accurately. This will be discussed in more detail in Chapter 7.

Complex family trees

Sometimes a family tree, where there is more than one individual affected by the same disorder, will show a pattern that is not compatible with a single-gene disorder. One possible explanation is that the affected individuals have the same disorder by chance rather than because of any shared genetic identity. This is particularly likely in common diseases such as cancer. About 1 in 3 people develop cancer during their lifetime. Most cancer is not inherited and the existence of two affected individuals in the same family is likely to occur by chance alone. Chapter 9 considers this in more detail.

It is also possible that there is more than one condition in the family and therefore it is important to verify from all possible sources the information on which any one disease has been

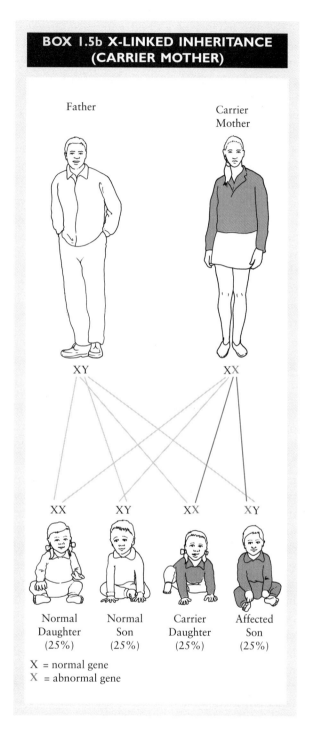

BOX 1.5a X-LINKED INHERITANCE (AFFECTED FATHER)

Affected Father

Mother

XY

XX

XX   XY   XX   XY

Carrier Daughter (25%)

Normal Son (25%)

Carrier Daughter (25%)

Normal Son (25%)

X = normal gene
X = abnormal gene

BOX 1.5b X-LINKED INHERITANCE (CARRIER MOTHER)

Father

Carrier Mother

XY

XX

XX   XY   XX   XY

Normal Daughter (25%)

Normal Son (25%)

Carrier Daughter (25%)

Affected Son (25%)

X = normal gene
X = abnormal gene

diagnosed. For example, hereditary haemorrhagic telangiectasia (HHT) is an autosomal dominant condition characterized by recurrent nosebleeds, mucocutaneous telangiectases (red spots on the lips and tongue, Fig. 1.5) and blood vessel abnormalities known as arteriovenous malformations. In a typical family tree of a patient with HHT there may well be a relative with recurrent nosebleeds whom the patient wrongly thinks is affected. Many individuals in the general population have recurrent nosebleeds and it is important to look for evidence of other, more specific, features of

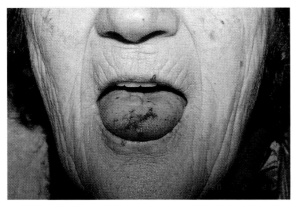

Fig. 1.5 Mutocutaneous telangiectases of the tongue found in hereditary haemorrhagic telangiectasia.

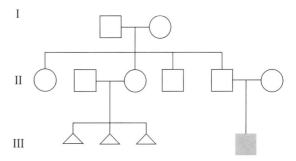

Fig. 1.6 Typical chromosome translocation family tree.

HHT such as telangiectases before accepting the diagnosis.

Chromosome translocations

Where the disorder in the family is due to a chromosome translocation (Chapter 2, **Box 2.3**) rather than a single-gene mutation, the family tree may be initially hard to interpret. Individuals carrying a balanced chromosome translocation are unaffected and may pass on either the normal chromosome pattern, a balanced translocation chromosome pattern, or an unbalanced chromosome translocation pattern. Clues to the presence of a translocation in a family tree include:

● recurrent miscarriages
● unexplained infertility
● mental handicap associated with an unusual or dysmorphic appearance in more than one individual related through phenotypically normal parents
● child or stillbirth with multiple malformations

The family tree outlined in Fig. 1.6 represents a typical family with a chromosome translocation. In this family individual II-3 has a poor obstetric history with three miscarriages. Her brother II-5 and his wife II-6 have a son III-1 with severe learning difficulties and a heart defect. His karyotype shows an unbalanced translocation. Analysis of his father's karyotype shows the balanced form of the same translocation. Individual II-3 shares the same balanced translocation as her brother. It is important that the translocation is traced as far as possible through the family so that individuals carrying the translocation can be informed of their risks. This concept is discussed in more detail in Case 2.3 in the next chapter.

Mitochondrial inheritance

Mammalian cells contain mitochondria which have their own circular deoxyribonucleic acid (DNA). Mitochondria are only passed on in the cytoplasm of the egg so that a child inherits all its mitochondria from its mother. There are some diseases that are associated with mutations in mitochondrial DNA. A woman with such a mutation will therefore pass it on to all her children whilst a man with the same mutation will not pass it on to any of his children. There is often a wide range of severity of disease in carriers of mitochondrial mutations.

Mitochondrial inheritance is characterized by:

● maternal transmission only
● extreme variability in the same family

PRINCIPLES OF GENETIC COUNSELLING

Genetic counselling has been defined as 'the process by which patients or relatives at risk of a disorder that may be hereditary are advised of the consequences of the disorder, the probability of developing or transmitting it and of the ways in which this may be prevented, avoided or ameliorated' (Professor P. Harper, see Further reading).

A key feature in this definition is the dissemination of information and so accurate information about the diagnosis and family structure is a vital component of the counselling process.

It is helpful to begin the session with a series of questions to be put directly to the consultand which will establish the agenda of the consultand.

- **Whose idea was the appointment?**
  - That of the consultand or the referring physician?
  - Is attendance at the genetic clinic compulsory before a particular procedure will be performed, e.g. reversal of sterilization, ovum donation?
- **What questions are you hoping to have answered?**
- **What have you been told already?**
  - Are there any misconceptions that need to be addressed?

Information should be given in a non-directive manner, i.e. without any bias introduced by the counsellor. This can be difficult when faced with questions such as 'what would you do?' Such a question may be deflected by suggesting possible alternatives, for example 'some people might do … what do you think about that?' If possible the consultand should be encouraged to repeat some of the information in his/her own words to confirm an understanding of the information. The session should be brought to an end with a summary of the information given and where possible followed up by a summary letter.

FURTHER READING

Bennett RL, Steinhaus KA, Uhrich SB, O'Sullivan CK, Resta RG, Lochner-Doyle D, Markel DS, Vincent V, Hamanishi J (1995) Recommendations for standardized human pedigree nomenclature. *American Journal of Human Genetics* 56:745–752.

Harper PS (1993) *Practical Genetic Counselling*, 4th edn. Butterworth Heinemann, Oxford.

QUESTIONS (ANSWERS ON PAGE 167)

Answer 'true' or 'false'.

1 In the family tree shown in Fig. 1.7

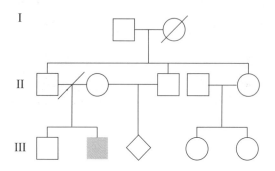

Fig. 1.7

- **a** I-2 is dead.
- **b** II-2 is male.
- **c** III-2 is affected.
- **d** III-1 and III-3 are a consanguineous couple.
- **e** II-3 has one boy.

2 In the family tree shown in Fig. 1.8

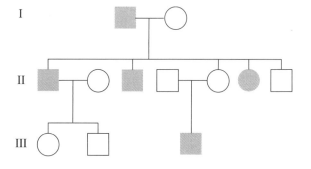

Fig. 1.8

- **a** The condition is X-linked.
- **b** II-5 is a non-penetrant gene carrier.
- **c** There is a 50% chance that any offspring of II-3 will carry the faulty gene.
- **d** The condition is likely to affect males and females equally.
- **e** III-1 and III-2 have 50% of their genes in common.

3 In the family tree shown in Fig. 1.9

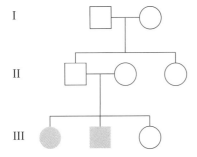

Fig. 1.9.

a The condition is autosomal recessive.
b There is a 2 out of 3 chance that II-1 and II-2 will have another affected child.
c III-3 has a 50% chance of being a carrier of the condition.
d III-1 and III-3 have 50% of their genes in common.
e I-1 and III-3 have 25% of their genes in common.

4 In the family tree shown in Fig. 1.10

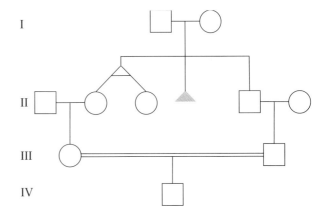

Fig. 1.10

a III-1 and III-2 are consanguineous.
b II-2 and II-3 are dizygotic twins.
c III-1 and III-2 have an increased risk of having a child with an autosomal dominant disorder.
d I-2 had a miscarriage of an affected fetus.
e II-2 and II-3 have 100% of their genes in common.

2

Chromosome Abnormalities

LEARNING OBJECTIVES

After studying this chapter, the reader should understand:

- the concept of a haploid and diploid genome
- the structure and description of human chromosomes
- the consequences of chromosome abnormality
- the importance of family studies in chromosome abnormalities
- the mechanisms of non-disjunction

INTRODUCTION

The 46 chromosomes (23 pairs) present in each human cell nucleus are stably inherited packages of double-stranded deoxyribonucleic acid (DNA) which store the genetic blueprint for all the inherited characteristics of an individual. Of these 46 the 22 autosomal pairs are numbered 1 to 22 in descending order of size. The remaining pair are called the sex chromosomes, which in females are two X chromosomes and in males are an X and a Y chromosome (Fig. 2.1). The presence of chromosome pairs implies that human cells require two copies of the DNA blueprint (also called the genome) for normal function; this is called a diploid genome. Each person inherits one chromosome in each pair from their mother and one from their father by fusion of haploid cells (i.e. cells containing only one copy of the genome).

- The egg cell contains 23 chromosomes = maternal genome
  - one of each autosome
  - one X chromosome
- The sperm contains 23 chromosomes = paternal genome
  - one of each autosome
  - one sex-determining chromosome (if the sperm carries an X chromosome the fertilized embryo will be female, or if it carries a Y chromosome a male embryo results).

Chromosomes are contained in the nucleus where they produce effects on other parts of the cell by acting as templates for the transcription of single-stranded ribonucleic acid (RNA) molecules. A transcribed chromosomal region that produces an effect in the cell is called a gene (see Chapter 3).

In 1956 the correct chromosome number in man was reported and 3 years later the first human chromosome anomalies were identified in Down syndrome and Klinefelter syndrome. Since that time with the tremendous advances in the analysis and description of chromosomes (**Box 2.1**) it has been found that chromosome abnormalities are very common in human populations. Approximately 8% of all clinically recognized pregnancies and 50% of spontaneous abortions have a chromosome abnormality. These are classified as numerical abnormalities (**Box 2.2**, Cases 2.2 and 2.3) and structural abnormalities (**Box 2.3**, Cases 2.4–2.6). Aneuploidy is a term for gain or loss of chromosome material compared with the normal constitution of the cell. In general, autosomal

(a)

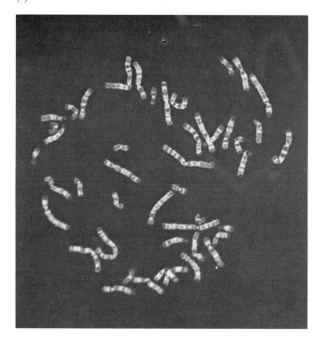

(b)

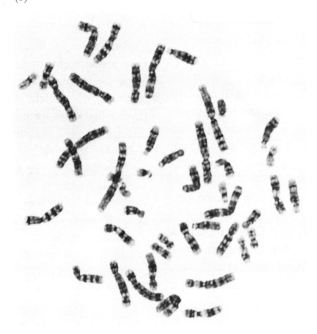

Fig. 2.1 The 46 human chromosomes. Normal female (a) and male (b) Giemsa-banded metaphase chromosomes as they would appear looking down a microscope. Chromosomes cut out from photographs of metaphase chromosome preparations and arranged into 23 homologous pairs in the female (c) and 22 homologous pairs and X and Y chromosomes in males (d). Note the position of the centromeric constriction along the length of the chromosomes dividing each into a short arm (p) and long arm (q). (Figure supplied by Mrs Elizabeth Grace.)

(c)

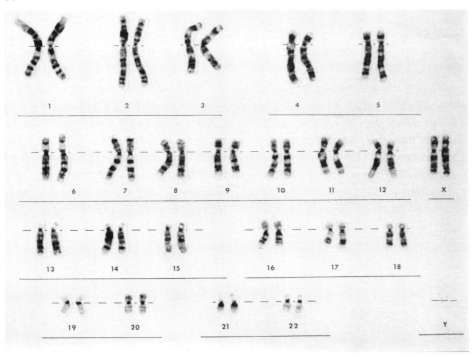

(d)

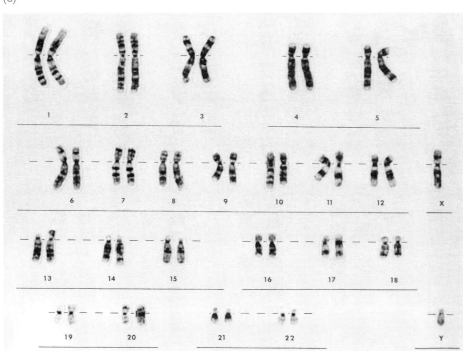

BOX 2.1 CHROMOSOME IDENTIFICATION AND ISCN

Human chromosomes are usually analysed by halting them in a specific stage of the cell cycle called metaphase (**Box 2.6**). In metaphase chromosomes have a constriction at one point along their length called a centromere. The centromere divides the chromosome into a long arm and a short arm. If the centromere is near the middle, the chromosome is called metacentric and if it is near the end it is called acrocentric. The ends of the chromosome arms are called the telomeres. In the early days of clinical chromosome analysis (also called clinical cytogenetics) chromosomes were described purely by their size and whether they were meta- or acrocentric. This was not satisfactory as not all the individual chromosomes could be definitively identified. Since the 1970s cytogenetic analysis has relied on various staining techniques to produce recognizable and reproducible banding patterns that can identify all human chromosomes (Fig. 2.1). There are many techniques that can be used to band chromosomes. However, the most frequently used in clinical cytogenetics is G-banding (Giemsa staining).

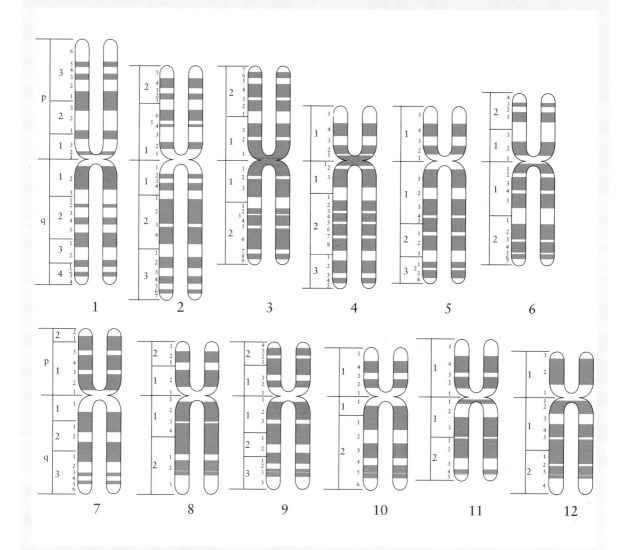

BOX 2.1 CHROMOSOME IDENTIFICATION AND ISCN (Cont.)

The use of banding meant that a standard way of describing chromosomes had to be developed and the main features of this International System for Cytogenetic Nomenclature (ISCN) are:

◆ the number of chromosomes in each cell is stated first; normally 46
◆ the complement of sex chromosomes is then stated; 46,XX for a female and 46,XY for a male
◆ the autosomal chromosome pairs are given a number from 1 to 22 (in descending order of size with chromosome 1 as the largest)

◆ extra or missing chromosomes can then be described easily, e.g. the karyotype of a male with three copies of chromosome 21 (Down syndrome) would be 47,XY,+21
◆ the short arm of any chromosome is labelled p (for petit) and the long arm q (the reverse of p)
◆ each band on a chromosome arm is assigned a number which gets larger the further the band is from the centromere, i.e. q13 is closer to the centromere than q27 (Fig. 2.2)

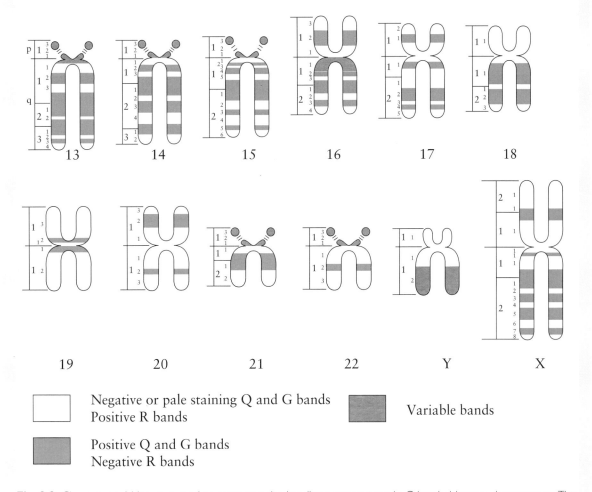

Negative or pale staining Q and G bands
Positive R bands

Variable bands

Positive Q and G bands
Negative R bands

Fig. 2.2 Chromosomal ideogram used to represent the banding patterns seen in G-banded human chromosomes. The numbers representing the bands increase from centromere to telomere. These chromosomes are represented as sister chromatids. (See Figure 2.4.) Q, G and R banding is explained in more detail in Box 2.8.

BOX 2.2 NUMERICAL CHROMOSOME ANOMALIES

Numerical abnormalities fall into four main categories (examples are given as a female karyotype):

◆ **trisomy** – an extra chromosome in each cell. The chromosomes that are found to be trisomic in live-born infants are 13 (47,XX,+13 Patau syndrome), 18 (46,XX+18 Edwards syndrome) and 21 (46,XX,+21 Down syndrome). Trisomies of all other chromosomes apart from 1 and 19 have been found in spontaneous abortions but are not normally compatible with late fetal development

◆ **monosomy** – a missing chromosome in each cell. Apart from monosomy of chromosome X in a female (45,X Turner syndrome) monosomy is rare in postnatal life

◆ **polyploidy** – extra set (69,XXX or 69,XXY, triploidy) or sets (92,XXXX tetraploidy) of total haploid genome

◆ **extra structurally abnormal chromosome (ESAC)** – also called additional marker chromosomes. These can be inherited with no clinical effect. The phenotype associated with ESAC depends on the precise nature of the genetic material involved: ~50% of all ESACs are inverted duplications of chromosome 15 derived material (see also **Box 2.5**, Pallister–Killian syndrome).

BOX 2.3 STRUCTURAL CHROMOSOME ANOMALIES

There are many different types of structural chromosome anomalies (examples are given as a female karyotype, Fig. 2.3):

◆ **deletions (del)** – absence of normal chromosomal material; can be terminal (removing an end of a chromosome) or interstitial. The missing part is described using the code 'del' followed by the number of the chromosome involved in brackets, followed by a description of the missing region of that chromosome in a separate set of brackets, e.g. 46,XX,del(1)(q21;qter) describes loss of the end of the long arm of chromosome 1. Some deletions result in clinically recognizable conditions associated with mental handicap:
  ◆ del(4p) – Wolf–Hirschhorn syndrome, unusual face with 'Greek-helmet' appearance
  ◆ del(5p) – cri du chat, unusual high-pitched cry.

◆ **duplications (dup)** – presence of an extra copy of a chromosomal segment; can be tandem or inverted:
  ◆ dup(22)(p13;q11) – cat-eye syndrome, iris coloboma.

◆ **inversions (inv)** – intrachromosomal re-arrangement such that the rearranged section is inverted; can be paracentric (does not include the centromere) or pericentric (includes the centromere).

◆ **ring chromosomes (r)** – deletion of the normal telomere (and possibly other subtelomeric sequences) with fusion of the ends to form a circular chromosome; often causes growth failure and mental handicap.

◆ **translocations** – interchromosomal rearrangement; can be balanced (the cell has a normal content of genetic material arranged in a structurally abnormal way) or unbalanced (the cell has gained or lost genetic material as a result of chromosomal interchange). Translocations can be reciprocal (Case 2.4) or Robertsonian (Case 2.5).

◆ **fragile sites (fra)** – are apparent gaps in a chromosome which can be divided into common (universal) or rare, folate-sensitive fragile sites. The latter are inherited in a Mendelian fashion and can be associated with disease (see Chapter 8, Fragile X syndrome)

BOX 2.3 STRUCTURAL CHROMOSOME ANOMALIES (Cont.)

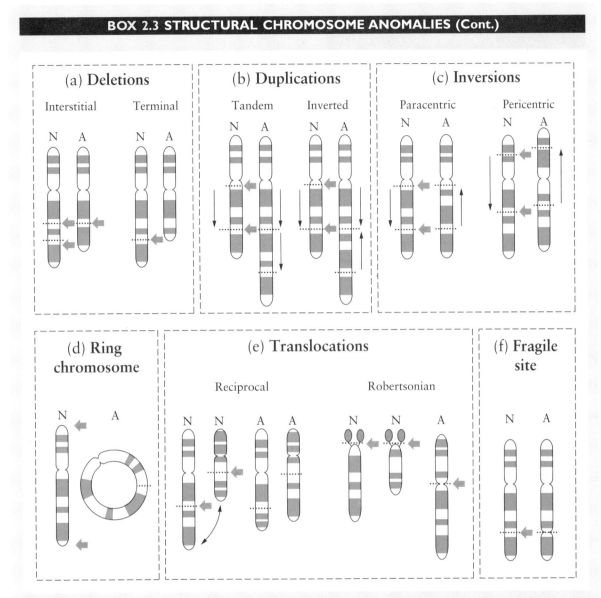

Fig. 2.3 An idealized chromosomal ideogram used to give examples of each structural chromosomal problem mentioned in the text: deletions (a), duplications (b), inversions (c), ring chromosomes (d), translocations (e) and fragile sites (f). N, normal chromosome; A, abnormal chromosome and grey arrow indicate breakpoint.

aneuploidy will have a profound negative effect on the physical and mental development of the affected individual. Aneuploidy of the sex chromosomes tends to have a less severe effect (**Box 2.4**). If present a chromosomal anomaly is usually observed in every cell studied in an individual. Where there are two or more cells found with different genetic constitutions in the same individual this is termed mosaicism (**Box 2.5**).

BOX 2.4 SEX CHROMOSOMAL ANOMALIES

◆ **Turner syndrome** – 45,X (Case 2.3).

◆ **Triple X syndrome** – 47,XXX, often asymptomatic, mild learning difficulties, tall slender body shape.

◆ **Klinefelter syndrome** – 47,XXY, infertility, small testes, hypogonadism, gynaecomastia, occasional mild learning problems.

◆ **47,XYY** – often asymptomatic, occasional behavioural problems.

◆ **46,XX males** – may result from the translocation of the sex-determining gene SRY from the Y chromosome onto the X chromosome via the short arm (pseudoautosomal) pairing seen in meiosis.

CASE 2.1
Chromosome analysis and heteromorphisms

Family tree

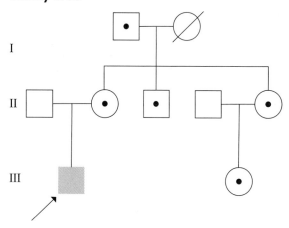

I

II

III

Presenting problem

A 4-year-old boy called Billy (III-1) with a bilateral cleft lip is seen by a local paediatrician for investigation of his mild mental handicap. She has sent a blood sample for chromosome analysis.

Why was chromosome analysis performed?

Mental handicap affects ~3% of children and has

BOX 2.5 CHROMOSOMAL MOSAICISM

Mosaicism describes the presence of different karyotypes found in a cell population that has arisen from one ancestral cell. This can cause problems in clinical settings since in some individuals the peripheral blood chromosomes may be normal whereas another tissue such as skin may show an abnormal karyotype. Some recognizable clinical conditions are caused by chromosome anomalies which have been described only in mosaic form because they are thought to be lethal if carried by all cells. Examples of this shown in a female karyotype are:

◆ **Turner syndrome** – many cases of Turner syndrome (see Case 3) are mosaic, e.g. 45,X/46,XX. Overall, sex chromosome abnormalities are the most common form of mosaicism seen in clinical practice.

◆ **Pallister-Killian syndrome** – 46,XX/ 47,XX,+iso(12p); iso(12p) is an extra structurally abnormal chromosome (ESAC see **Box 2.2**) comprising two copies of the short arm of chromosome 12. The cells that contain the iso(12p) thus have four copies of 12p (tetrasomy 12p). This leads to severe mental handicap, unusual facies and areas of skin hypopigmentation.

◆ **Mosaic trisomy 8** – 46,XX/47,XX,+8, tall stature, mental retardation, unusual groove in sole of foot.

many causes (**Box 2.6**). Analysis of chromosomes in a clinical cytogenetics laboratory is a standard test in this situation since abnormalities in the number or structure of human chromosomes often result in both mental and physical handicap. The test is carried out by a clinical cytogeneticist who analyses human chromosomes using a light microscope. Most chromosome analysis in children and adults is done using peripheral blood lymphocytes (**Box 2.7**) although dividing cells from any tissue can be used.

BOX 2.6 CAUSES OF MENTAL HANDICAP

Approximately 3% of all children born will have significant intellectual handicap; some of the more common causes of mental retardation are given below. This is a rough estimate and the proportions in different categories will vary with the severity of the handicap.

◆ **Genetic causes**
  ◆ chromosome abnormalities ~10%
  ◆ single gene abnormalities ~15% (a significant proportion of these have Fragile X syndrome)
  ◆ identifiable syndrome diagnoses ~5%
◆ **Environmental causes**
  ◆ teratogens (environmental agents causing damage before birth) 1%
  ◆ 'birth injury' 12%
  ◆ childhood infections (meningitis, encephalitis) ~7%
◆ **Unknown aetiology** ~50%

What was the result?

Analysis of Giemsa-banded (G-banded) chromosomes showed that on one of Billy's chromosome 6 there was a large extra piece of material near the middle of the chromosome (Fig. 2.5). This was reported as 46,XY,var(6q). Further study in the family showed that the same unusual chromosome was present in his mother and also in his uncle, aunt, cousin and grandfather on his mother's side of the family.

Is the variant chromosome causing the handicap?

In general, there is little or no difference in the appearance of G-banded chromosomes between individuals. Since Billy inherited this from his mother, who is of normal intelligence, and it has also been found in other normal members of his extended family, it is extremely unlikely to have anything to do with Billy's mental handicap. Therefore the chromosomal anomaly found in this family is a heteromorphism or benign inherited variant chromosome.

BOX 2.7 CHROMOSOME ANALYSIS

For standard cytogenetic analysis, the presence of actively dividing cells is necessary. Blood lymphocytes must, therefore, be stimulated to divide using a chemical mitogen. The mitotic cell cycle is divided into five stages (Fig. 2.4):

◆ **G_0 or interphase** – chromosomes are long and thread-like (decondensed)
◆ **G_1** – increase in metabolic activity
◆ **S** – DNA synthesis and chromosomal replication which results in a 'double' chromosome joined at the centromere (sister chromatids)
◆ **G_2** – formation of spindle apparatus and chromosome condensation begins
◆ **M or metaphase** – cell division with chromosome condensed

By adding a chemical blocker, such as colchicine, it is possible to arrest the cell cycle at the stage of chromatin condensation in G_2 and M phase. Condensed chromosomes can then be stained to produce banding patterns (Fig. 2.2). Techniques vary slightly between laboratories but a typical protocol is shown below:

◆ Add whole blood to culture medium with phytohaemagglutinin (PHA) (mitogen stimulating lymphocytes to divide).
◆ Incubate for 70 h.
◆ Add a mitotic spindle inhibitor such as colchicine which introduces a block between metaphase and anaphase and culture for 2 h.
◆ Collect cells by centrifugation, lyse cells in hypotonic solution and collect nuclei by centrifugation.
◆ Fix nuclei in methanol/acetic acid mixture.
◆ Drop onto glass slides, stain and analyse under light microscope.

BOX 2.7 CHROMOSOME ANALYSIS (Cont.)

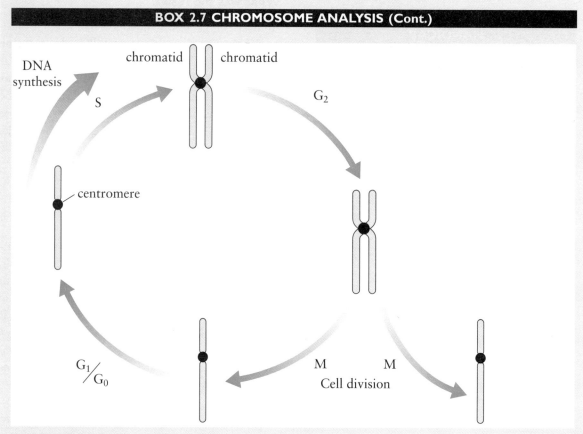

Fig. 2.4 When a non-dividing (G_0 stage) cell, or a cell which has completed a previous division (a G_1 stage cell), begins to divide, it first enters the S phase (DNA synthesis). During S phase, the double-stranded DNA replicates to yield two identical double-stranded molecules. These are held together at the centromere with mitosis (M phase), and are called sister chromatids. At cell division (mitosis, M phase) the centromere splits and the sister chromatids enter separate daughter cells.

What is the extra material on chromosome 6?

Using a staining method called 'C' banding (**Box 2.8**) the extra material at the centromere stained darkly showing it is comprised of constitutive heterochromatin. Constitutive heterochromatin has no known genetic function. Therefore, considerable differences in the size of these regions can be tolerated by the cell with no ill effects. In contrast, it is very unusual to have any normal variation in the light staining bands (euchromatin) in which most of the important genetic information is concentrated. Without investigating the family the chromosome result in Billy could have been misinterpreted as the cause of his handicap. Common heteromorphisms involve chromosomes 1, 9, 16, Y and acrocentric chromosomes.

CASE 2.2
Down syndrome caused by chromosomal non-disjunction

Family Tree

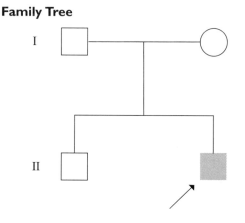

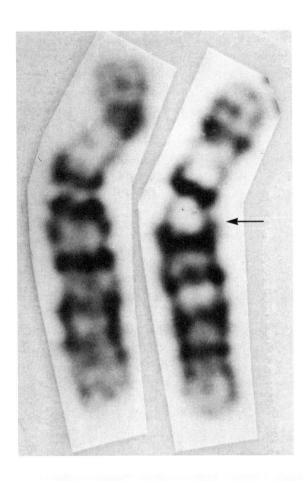

Fig. 2.5 Billy's chromosome analysis showing an unusual pattern on one chromosome 6q (arrowed). Exactly the same pattern was found in several unaffected relatives.

Presenting problem

John (II-2) is 19 months old. He was born at 40 weeks' gestation weighing 2830 g after an uneventful pregnancy. At birth he was noted to be a very floppy baby and an experienced midwife, within half an hour of birth, alerted the paediatric team that she thought John had Down syndrome. On examination he was found to have a cardiac murmur which was later shown to be due to a ventricular septal defect. This required no treatment and further investigations revealed no other major malformations. John's mother, Jessica, is now 8 weeks pregnant.

What alerted the midwife to the diagnosis in John?

The midwife noticed that John had certain facial features which are characteristic of Down syndrome (Fig. 2.6); upslanting palpebral fissures, a flat nasal bridge and mid-face, a small mouth, small ears, Brushfield spots (a white speckling of

BOX 2.8 STRUCTURE OF METAPHASE CHROMOSOMES

DNA is negatively charged and in metaphase chromosomes it is associated with various anionic metals, polyamines and proteins. The most abundant of the proteins are known as histones. DNA coils round a complex of five different histones to form a structure, named chromatin. This is the first level of a remarkable, chromosomal condensation mechanism. This condensation or 'reeling-in' mechanism means that although an average human chromosome is ~4.4 cm long as a native DNA strand, its length at its most condensed stage during metaphase is only ~6 μm. This represents a ~73 000-fold reduction in length.

Chromosome bands are variations in longitudinal structure of the chromatin demonstrated by various staining techniques. The major band types are:

◆ **C-bands.** These are regions of centromeric constitutive heterochromatin containing tandemly repeated segments of DNA and with no apparent genetic function (see Case 2.1).

◆ **Quinacrine- (Q-bands) or Giemsa-dark bands.** DNA sequences use a code with only four elements or bases: adenine (A), guanine (G), cytosine (C) and thymine (T). The DNA sequences which form Q-bands contain a higher proportion of A and T bases (AT-rich) but contain only ~20% of mapped human genes.

◆ **Reverse- (R-bands) or Giemsa-pale bands.** These contain a higher proportion of C and G bases (CG-rich) and contain almost all widely expressed human genes. Any abnormality in these euchromatic regions usually causes a severe clinical phenotype.

◆ **Nucleolar organizer regions (NOR).** NOR contain the highly active genes for the 18S and 28S ribosomal RNA (rRNA) and are located in the short arms of the acrocentric human chromosomes (chromosomes 13, 14, 15, 21 and 22).

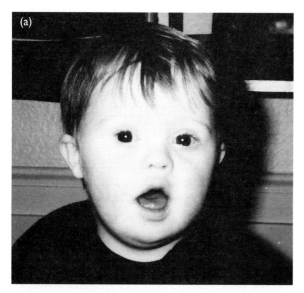

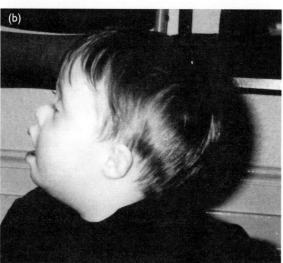

Fig. 2.6 The facial appearance of a child with Down syndrome from the front (a) and from the left side (b).

the iris) and brachycephaly (flattening of the occiput making the head look unusually round). In addition to the facial features his hands show brachydactyly (shortening of the digits) and a single transverse palmar crease. His feet show a large gap between the first and second toe bilaterally (see Chapter 6, Fig. 6.3).

What is the cause of Down syndrome?

Down syndrome is caused by the presence of three copies of part or all of chromosome 21. Chromosome analysis in John's case showed a male karyotype with an additional chromosome 21 in each cell (47,XY,+21). Ninety-five per cent of cases of Down syndrome are due to the presence of trisomy 21 (i.e. 47,XX,+21 or 47,XY,+21). However, Down syndrome can also be caused by a translocation (see Case 2.5) or, rarely, a duplication (**Box 2.3**) involving 21q22.2 known as the Down syndrome critical region (DCR), trisomy of which appears to be responsible for most of the characteristic features of Down syndrome.

How did the extra chromosome 21 arise?

The extra copy of chromosome 21 in each of John's cells must have arisen by a process of abnormal segregation (sorting) of chromosomes during cell division, called non-disjunction. Non-disjunction can occur either during the production of egg and sperm cells or in the first few divisions of the fertilized egg. The former is meiotic non-disjunction and the latter post-zygotic mitotic (PZM) non-disjunction (see **Box 2.9**). There are two types of meiotic non-disjunction:

● errors which occur in first meiotic (MI), or
● errors which occur in second meiotic (MII) cell division (Fig. 2.7).

Most cases of Down syndrome occur as a result of non-disjunction in MI. The extra 21 in Down syndrome is maternal in origin in 91% of cases and paternal in 9%. The cause of non-disjunction is not known but it becomes more common with maternal age (**Box 2.10**).

What does the future hold for John?

John was noted to be significantly slower in all aspects of his development as compared with his unaffected sibling. He had no other major malformations associated with Down syndrome although he is as yet too young for the later onset clinical problems associated with Down syndrome (**Box 2.11**).

Life expectancy in people with Down syndrome is improving and now is >60 years in the absence of serious malformations. Most people with Down syndrome do not have children due to the intellectual handicap and the fact that males appear to be infertile while females have reduced fertility.

BOX 2.9 NON-DISJUNCTION

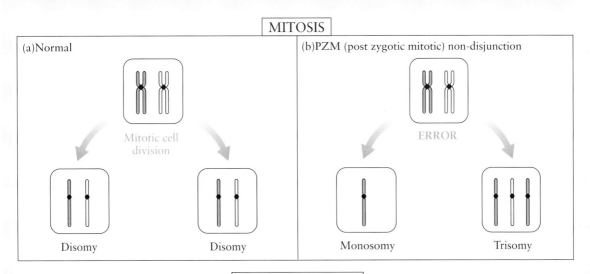

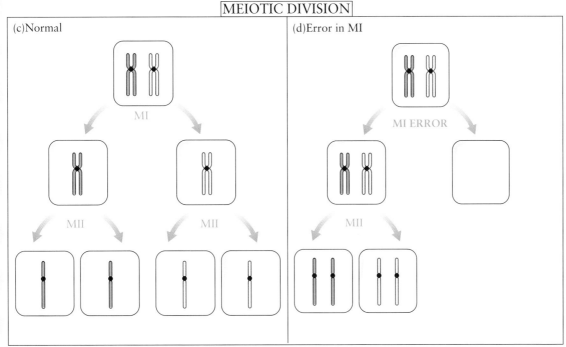

Fig. 2.7 Chromosome segregation during normal cell division and non-disjunction. Normal mitosis (a) involves the replication of each chromosome to produce two identical chromatids joined at the centromere. These chromatids are pulled into different poles of the cell resulting in two daughter cells each with 46 chromosomes. In PZM non-disjunction (b) both sister chromatids from one chromosome are pulled into one pole resulting in one daughter cell with 47 chromosomes (trisomy) and one with 45 (monosomy). Normal meiosis (c) is more complicated. Prior to MI (first meiotic cell division), DNA replication occurs resulting in a cell with 46 chromosomes (92 chromatids). After MI each daughter cell has 23 chromosomes (46 chromatids) and after MII each daughter cell has 23 chromosomes (23 chromatids). Non-disjunction errors in MI (d) and MII (e) both result in daughter cells that are multisomic (no chromosome present) and disomic for a particular chromosome.

BOX 2.9 NON-DISJUNCTION (Cont.)

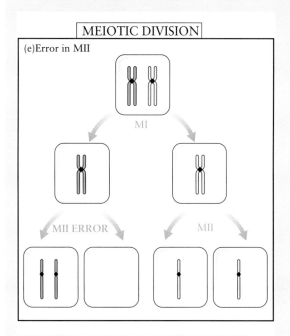

Both egg cells and sperm cells are formed by a germline specific cellular process called meiosis (Fig. 2.7c). The purpose of meiotic cell divisions is to create haploid germ cells in the male and female gonad. This is achieved by having two rounds of cell division, meiosis I (MI) and meiosis II (MII), with only one phase of

chromosome replication (prior to MI). At the end of MII each cell has 23 chromosomes (one copy of each autosome and a sex chromosome). Prior to MI, the two chromosomes of a homologous pair become closely associated along their whole length, which allows the exchange of genetic material between the maternally and paternally derived chromosomes. These chromosomal exchange events in meiosis are very important throughout clinical genetics and will be discussed in more detail in Chapter 4.

Both the timing and cellular processes of meiosis are different in males and females. In the testes meiotic division begins at puberty and continues throughout life. In females meiosis is much more prolonged, beginning towards the end of intrauterine life in the fetal ovary. The process then arrests prior to MI and is completed only after puberty prior to each ovulation. MI in maturing oocytes does not produce two daughter cells but one daughter cell and the first polar body containing 23 inactive chromosomes (46 chromatids). A second meiotic arrest then occurs until fertilization at which time MII occurs producing the second polar body and the female pronucleus which will fuse with the male pronucleus released from the sperm head.

However, the risk of any offspring of an affected parent also having Down syndrome is ~50%.

What are the chances that John's mother's current pregnancy will be affected?

If a young woman has a pregnancy affected with Down syndrome then there is an increased chance of recurrence in a future pregnancy. This risk is 0.5–1% for each pregnancy. In women >40 years old the risk of recurrence in future pregnancies does not appear to be significantly different from the age-related risk. Fetal karyotyping is currently the only way to be sure whether or not a pregnancy is affected. This is performed on cells obtained at amniocentesis or by chorionic villus sampling (see Chapter 6).

CASE 2.3
Turner syndrome

Family tree

BOX 2.10 FEATURES OF NON-DISJUNCTION OF CHROMOSOME 21

◆ Down syndrome occurs in all human populations at approximately the same rate (~1 case in every 600 births) and is unlikely to be related to any specific environmental factors.
◆ There is a significant loss of trisomy 21 embryos via spontaneous abortion in early pregnancy and it has been estimated that as many as 1 in 150 clinically recognized pregnancies have trisomy 21.
◆ The risk of having a pregnancy affected with Down syndrome is closely related to the maternal but not to the paternal age; the mother's age-related risk is:
  ◆ 1:2000 at age 20
  ◆ 1:1000 at age 30
  ◆ 1:110 at age 40

BOX 2.11 CLINICAL ASSOCIATIONS WITH DOWN SYNDROME

Congenital malformations
◆ **Congenital heart defects** – 40%
  ◆ atrioventricular septal defect
  ◆ ventricular septal defect
  ◆ atrial septal defect
◆ **Duodenal atresia** – 3-5%

Late-onset clinical problems
  ◆ a non-specific immunodeficiency with particular susceptibility to respiratory infections
  ◆ a significantly increased risk of leukaemia (~15–20 × greater than other children)
  ◆ a susceptibility to dementia similar to Alzheimer's disease

Presenting problem

Alice (II-1) is a healthy 14-year-old girl being investigated by the paediatric endocrinologist for short stature; her height is below the 3rd centile for chronological age (see Chapter 10, Fig. 10.1). A routine chromosome analysis showed a 45,X karyotype and a diagnosis of Turner syndrome was

made. On clinical examination Alice had none of the other physical anomalies associated with 45,X (**Box 2.12**). However, on pelvic ultrasound she was found to have abnormally small ovaries bilaterally.

BOX 2.12 FEATURES OF TURNER SYNDROME

Physical features
◆ short stature
◆ webbing of the neck
◆ coarctation (narrowing) of the aorta
◆ perinatal oedema (puffiness) of hands and feet
◆ increased carrying angle at the elbow
Other features
◆ normal intelligence
◆ ovaries may appear normal at birth with progressive atrophy throughout childhood. This may be because during oogenesis a double dose of X genes may be required; the ovary is the only tissue where reversal of X-inactivation occurs
◆ ~99% of fetuses with 45,X karyotype are spontaneously aborted in early pregnancy
◆ other karyotypes can result in Turner syndrome including 46,X,iso(Xq) and 45,X/46,XX or 45,X/46,XY mosaicism
◆ it is thought that mosaicism for Y sequences in Turner syndrome results in an increased risk of developing gonadoblastoma

What is Turner syndrome?

Turner syndrome is monosomy of the X chromosome in females. Chromosomal monosomy, like trisomy, occurs as a result of non-disjunction. 45,X is the only monosomy compatible with postnatal life. In Turner syndrome it is most often the paternal X chromosome which is lost. It has puzzled geneticists for many years why having only one X chromosome should cause any clinical problems, since all women undergo X-inactivation (**Box 2.13**) and thus like men, have only one active X chromosome in each cell. The answer to this came with the discovery that there is a requirement for two copies of the few genes which escape X-inactivation.

BOX 2.13 X-INACTIVATION

Female embryos at about the 100 cell stage undergo a process called X inactivation or Lyonization. This is the transcriptional silencing (or genetic inactivation) of one of the pair of X chromosomes in each cell. The decision whether to switch off the X chromosome inherited from the mother or the X chromosome inherited from the father is random and, on average, 50% of cells will switch off one and 50% of cells will switch off the other. The result of this process is that women, like men, have only one active copy of the X chromosome in each cell. The inactive X chromosome in each cell condenses and can sometimes be seen as a dark staining body (Barr body or X-chromatin body) at the periphery of the nucleus (see Chapter 7, Box 7.1).

What are the clinical implications of Turner syndrome?

Growth hormone treatment has been successfully used to improve final adult height. Because there is primary ovarian failure most women with Turner syndrome require oestrogen supplementation to initiate and sustain normal pubertal development. Infertility is almost universal in Turner syndrome. However, since the uterus is normal in women with Turner syndrome, implantation of a donor egg fertilized *in vitro* has resulted in successful pregnancies.

Why do all men not get the malformations seen in Turner syndrome?

When an X chromosome is inactivated almost all the genes on that chromosome are switched off. However, a few genes escape X inactivation and it is thought that two active copies of these genes are required for normal development. At least some of these genes are in small regions present on the short arms of the X and Y chromosomes called the pseudoautosomal regions (Chapter 7, Box 7.2). Thus men do not develop the malformations seen in Turner syndrome because the pseudoautosomal

region on Yp also contains copies of the genes that escape X inactivation in the female. For normal development both men and women, therefore, require two active copies of a subset of X genes which are deficient in Turner syndrome.

CASE 2.4
Reciprocal translocation

Family tree

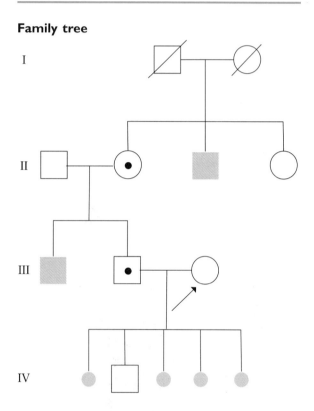

Presenting problem

Sheila (III-3) was referred by her obstetrician after four of her five pregnancies had ended in early spontaneous miscarriage. She has one normal son aged 4. Her husband, Scott (III-2), is in good health. His brother, Stephen (III-1), and maternal uncle, Philip (II-3), have severe physical and mental handicap. Sheila and Scott wished to know if there is a genetic cause for their miscarriages and their obstetrician sent blood samples for chromosome analysis on both of them which were reported as:

- Sheila 46,XX
- Scott 46,XY,t(1;15)(q21;p13)

Further investigations in the family revealed that Scott's father, Harry (II-1), has normal chromosomes and his mother, Patricia (II-2), has an identical autosomal pattern to Scott (her karyotype was 46,XX,t(1;15)(q21;p13)). Stephen and Philip were both found to have the karyotype 46,XY,der(15), t(1;15)(q21;p13).

What is this chromosomal abnormality?

Scott and his mother carry a balanced reciprocal translocation which involves an exchange of chromosomal material between chromosomes 1 and 15 (Box 2.3). The rearranged chromosomes are called derivative (der) chromosomes and these are named der(1) and der(15) according to which centromere they possess. The band on the chromosome where the chromosomal exchange has occurred is called the translocation breakpoint. Approximately 1 in 600 people in the population carry a balanced translocation which may involve exchange between any two or more chromosomes. Reciprocal translocations are, in many cases, inherited from one or other parent but can occur *de novo* (not present in either parent). *De novo* reciprocal translocations arise as a result of errors in parental meiosis.

What is the significance of a balanced translocation in an individual?

In the most cases balanced translocations do not cause any medical problems to the carrier. However, in some rare cases the translocation breakpoint may disrupt a specific gene. This has helped in the identification of the chromosomal location of genes involved in several genetic disorders (**Box 2.14**). Carriers of balanced translocations may have reproductive health problems such

---

BOX 2.14 RECIPROCAL TRANSLOCATIONS CAN AID THE IDENTIFICATION OF GENES

Most balanced reciprocal translocations cause no health problems in the carriers. Rarely, translocation breakpoints can disrupt a gene, causing an abnormal phenotype in the carrier. These families can be extremely helpful in the identification of genes mutated in particular phenotypes as it is now relatively simple to isolate the DNA sequences involved in translocation breakpoints. Below are listed some of the autosomal genes that have been localized or isolated with the help of reciprocal translocation breakpoints.

- neurofibromatosis type I (17q11.2)
- Greig cephalopolysyndactyly syndrome (7p13)
- aniridia (11p13)
- de Lange syndrome (3q26.1)
- blepharophimosis, epicanthus inversus and ptosis (3q23)

Another form of reciprocal translocation, X-autosome translocations, is particularly useful in gene mapping. In this situation chromosomal material is swapped between the X-chromosome and one of the autosomes. Females with these translocations inactivate the normal X chromosome in each cell because inactivation of the derivative X chromosome would result in loss of autosomal function and thus have a profound negative effect on cellular function. However, inactivating the normal X chromosome means that if the translocation breakpoint interrupts a gene on the X chromosome then the female may develop an X-linked recessive disease usually only seen in males (**Box 2.13** and Chapter 7). Some examples of this are:

- hypohidrotic ectodermal dysplasia 46,X,t(X;9)(q13.1;p24)
- Lowe oculocerebrorenal syndrome 46,X,t(X;3)(q25;q27)
- Norrie disease 46,X, t(X;10)(p11;p14)
- Duchenne muscular dystrophy 46,X,t(X,1)(p21;q31)

Reciprocal translocations can also occur as a somatic events which produce activation of genes involved in the multistep process of cancer development (Chapter 9, Box 9.3).

(a) Normal meiosis

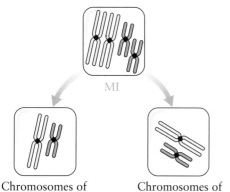

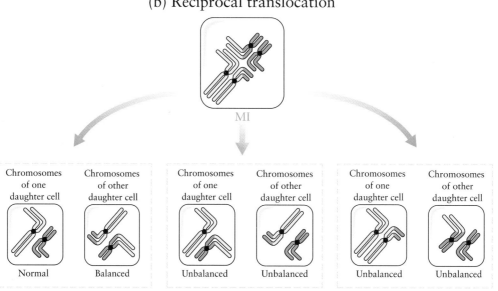

MI

Chromosomes of
one daughter cell

Chromosomes of
other daughter cell

Fig. 2.8 Association of homologous chromosomes prior to MI in chromosomally normal cells (a) and those with reciprocal (b) or Robertsonian (c) translocations. Homologous chromosomes are shaded in the same colour.

(b) Reciprocal translocation

MI

Chromosomes of one daughter cell	Chromosomes of other daughter cell	Chromosomes of one daughter cell	Chromosomes of other daughter cell	Chromosomes of one daughter cell	Chromosomes of other daughter cell
Normal	Balanced	Unbalanced	Unbalanced	Unbalanced	Unbalanced

(c) Robertsonian Translocation

MI

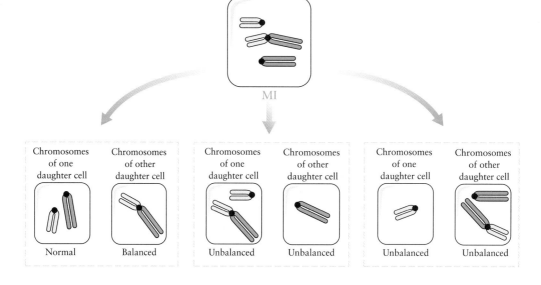

Chromosomes of one daughter cell	Chromosomes of other daughter cell	Chromosomes of one daughter cell	Chromosomes of other daughter cell	Chromosomes of one daughter cell	Chromosomes of other daughter cell
Normal	Balanced	Unbalanced	Unbalanced	Unbalanced	Unbalanced

as infertility, recurrent miscarriages and offspring with physical and mental disabilities. These problems result from abnormal segregation of derivative chromosomes during meiosis. Prior to the first meiotic division (MI) and after DNA replication homologous chromosomes become closely associated. In reciprocal translocations four of the chromosomes cannot pair completely. In this case it is chromosomes 1, 15, der(1) and der(15). To enable meiosis to proceed these four chromosomes must form a complex structure and segregation of these chromosomes into the daughter cells can lead to either chromosomally balanced or unbalanced gametes (Figs 2.8a, b).

While Scott inherited a balanced chromosomal complement from his mother as a der(1) and der(15), his brother inherited a normal chromosome 1 and der(15) which results in him being monosomic for a region of chromosome 15 and trisomic for a region of chromosome 1. This chromosomal imbalance has resulted in severe mental and physical handicap. The other form of unbalanced gamete, containing der(1) and normal chromosome 15 resulting in partial monosomy of chromosome 1 and partial trisomy of chromosome 15, has not been observed in this family. This is probably because this chromosome constitution is not compatible with late fetal development and results in a miscarriage.

What is the risk in this family in future pregnancies?

After the last miscarriage Sheila was seen in the genetics clinic and was told that there was a significant risk, probably greater than 10%, of having a child with a severe chromosome imbalance and also a high risk of having a pregnancy that would result in an early spontaneous miscarriage. Sheila decided to be sterilized as she felt she could not cope with further pregnancies. Her son, Stuart (IV-1), was not tested to see if he is a carrier for the translocation as he is healthy and under 16 years old. Children under the age of 16 are not usually tested unless the information is of direct medical relevance during childhood. Finally, an attempt has been made to contact other members of Patricia's

family so that they can be offered a test to identify other translocation carriers and make them aware of the possible reproductive risks.

CASE 2.5
Robertsonian translocation

Family tree

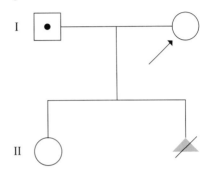

Presenting problem

Jane became pregnant for the second time at the age of 38 years. This pregnancy had occurred after a prolonged period of infertility. She and her husband James had decided to have an amniocentesis (see Chapter 6, Box 6.3) because of the age-related risk of Down syndrome (**Box 2.10**). Analysis of amniocytes has shown the karyotype 46,XY,−15, +rob(13;15). James was found to have a 45,XY, −13,−15,+rob(13;15) karyotype whilst Jane's chromosomes were normal. After discussing these results at 19 weeks of gestation they decided to terminate the pregnancy. A post-mortem examination of the fetus revealed multiple malformations (**Box 2.15**) and evidence of maceration suggesting that intrauterine death had occurred prior to the termination of pregnancy.

What would have been the likely outcome of this pregnancy?

This fetus was affected with Patau syndrome or trisomy 13. Karyotype 46,XY,−15,+rob(13;15) implies a male fetus with one chromosome 15 missing and replaced with a Robertsonian translocation involving chromosomes 13 and 15. This results in each cell being disomic for chromosome 15 and trisomic for chromosome 13. This chromosome constitution has characteristic clinical features (**Box 2.15**) and, if the pregnancy survives to term, is usually fatal within 3 months of birth.

BOX 2.15 CLINICAL FEATURES OF TRISOMY 13

- growth retardation
- holoprosencephaly
- cleft lip and palate
- cardiac malformations
- polydactyly
- kidney malformation
- defects in scalp
- fetal death

How do Robertsonian translocations arise?

Robertsonian translocations occur by centric fusion of the long arms of acrocentric chromosomes (chromosomes 13, 14, 15, 21 and 22). These can occur heterologously (between different chromosomes, e.g. rob(14;21)) or homologously (within a chromosome pair, e.g. rob(21;21)) with the former being much more common. In total, Robertsonian translocations occur in ~1 : 900 people with rob(13;14) as the most common. The chromosome number in carriers of balanced Robertsonian translocations is 45 rather than 46.

How did the trisomy 13 arise?

Most cases of trisomy 13 arise as a result of meiotic non-disjunction. However, in this case the trisomy has arisen as a result of abnormal segregation of a Robertsonian translocation during meiosis. In Robertsonian translocation carriers, as in reciprocal translocation carriers, chromosome pairing at meiosis is complex (Fig. 2.8c). However in Robertsonian translocations this involves three chromosomes rather than four. A proportion of the gametes will be aneuploid. In some male Robertsonian translocation carriers there is a block in MI during spermatogenesis causing a low sperm count. It may be that this is the cause of Jane and James' prolonged infertility.

What are the recurrence risks in a future pregnancy?

If Jane and James decide to have further pregnancies it may be predicted that a significant number of gametes would be chromosomally unbalanced and may result in a high frequency of pregnancies affected with trisomy 13 (trisomy 15 is not normally viable). However, in practice this is not observed as the risk of trisomy 13 in a future pregnancy is low (<1%) in carriers of t(13;15) and other Robertsonian translocations (**Box 2.16**). There appears to be some selection in both male and female meiosis against the unbalanced segregations, although this is more pronounced in males. It is not known how this is achieved.

BOX 2.16 RISK OF TRISOMY IN ROBERTSONIAN TRANSLOCATIONS

Rob(13;14) accounts for ~70% of all balanced Robertsonian translocations and rob(14;21) for ~15% and thus these are the only ones where good data on the risk of unbalanced offspring is available (see Table 2.1). Rob(21;22) is rare although it appears to have a relatively high risk of Down syndrome offspring in female carriers. Robertsonian translocations are responsible for <5% of Down syndrome. Homologous Robertsonian translocations such as rob(13;13) and rob(21;21) occur but are extremely rare and provide examples of the few situations where there is a 100% genetic risk of affected offspring.

Table 2.1 Risk of unbalanced offspring

Translocation	Risk of Trisomy in Offspring of Female Carriers (%)	Risk of Trisomy in Offspring of Male Carriers (%)
rob(13;14)	<1	<1
rob(14;21)	15	<1
rob(21;22)	10	5
rob(13;13)	100	100
rob(21;21)	100	100

CASE 2.6
Microdeletion of 22q11

Family tree

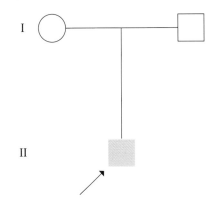

Presenting problem

Jamie was born at 37 weeks' gestation weighing 2930 g. He was well until day 3 when he became 'jittery' and was found to have a low plasma calcium level. On transfer to the neonatal unit he was noted to have a cardiac murmur and unusual facial features. The clinical geneticist was asked to see him and made the diagnosis of Di George syndrome (DGS). DGS is a combination of absent thymus, heart defects, hypocalcaemia caused by hypoparathyroidism and unusual facial features. Jamie had micrognathia (small jaw) and unusually shaped ears but otherwise did not have any external malformations. Cardiac ultrasound showed a tetralogy of Fallot defect (ventricular septal defect, pulmonary stenosis, over-riding aorta and ventricular hypertrophy) and the normal thymic shadow was absent on a neonatal chest X-ray. Chromosome analysis showed an apparently normal 46,XY karyotype, whereas fluorescent *in situ* hybridization (FISH) analysis (**Box 2.17**, Fig. 2.10) revealed a chromosomal microdeletion on 22q11. Both parents had normal karyotypes with no deletion of 22q11 on FISH analysis.

What is the cause of Di George syndrome?

Jamie has a microdeletion of chromosome 22q11, which is the cause of most cases of DGS. Microdeletions are regions of chromosomal loss which cannot be detected by routine cytogenetics. The resolution of light microscopy in cytogenetics is ~4 million base pairs of DNA, so any deletion smaller than this cannot be identified using conventional techniques. The advent of molecular cytogenetics has made the diagnosis of these deletions much easier (**Box 2.17**). It is not known what function genes in the deleted region fulfil in normal development, but they may affect a particular group of embryonic cells called neural crest cells (Chapter 10, Box 10.6). Microdeletions have been identified as the cause of a number of different clinical conditions (**Box 2.18**).

What does this diagnosis mean for Jamie and his parents?

Unfortunately, Jamie's prognosis is not good. The problems with DGS are not limited to the cardiac defect as the aplasia (failure to form) of the thymus results in a specific immunodeficiency, resulting in the child being highly susceptible to infections. A significant proportion of children with DGS die in the first year of life.

For Jamie's parents as the deletion has occurred *de novo* (i.e. not present in parents) the recurrence risk in a future pregnancy is low. However, there is a possibility that one of the parents could be a mosaic for the deletion so a recurrence risk of ~1% is often given (Chapter 8).

FURTHER READING

Gardiner RJM, Sutherland GR (1989) *Chromosome Abnormalities and Genetic Counselling.* OUP, Oxford.

Jacobs PA, Hassold TJ (1995) The origins of numerical chromosome anomalies. *Advances in Genetics* **33**: 101–133.

Saitoh Y, Laemmli UK (1994) Metaphase chromosome structure: Bands arise from a differential folding path of the highly AT-rich scaffold. *Cell* **76**: 609–622.

Schinzel A (1989) *Human Cytogenetics Database.* OUP, Oxford.

BOX 2.17 MOLECULAR CYTOGENETICS

Over the past 10 years several techniques have been developed to extend and facilitate cytogenetic analysis. The ability to generate DNA probes carrying a fluorescent label and hybridize specifically to known chromosomal regions has revolutionized clinical and research applications of cytogenetics. These techniques are generally known as fluorescence *in situ* hybridization (FISH). FISH has many applications including:

◆ chromosome painting – when the DNA probes used hybridize to the entire length of one chromosome pair (Fig. 2.9). This can be particularly useful in chromosomal analysis of cancers where the individual chromosomes may undergo complex rearrangements. Painting is also useful to identify genetic material in ESACs (**Box 2.2**).

◆ locus-specific metaphase FISH – this can be used to localize a gene to a chromosomal region or to look for submicroscopic deletions or duplications (Fig. 2.10; see Case 2.6)

◆ interphase FISH – this uses locus-specific probes to investigate the presence and physical spacing of particular chromosomal regions. Cell culture is not required prior to analysis and the technique can be used for the rapid identification of trisomies and chromosomal sex on prenatal samples (Fig. 2.11).

◆ comparative genomic hybridization (CGH) – this technique involves labelling with different colours the genomic DNA from two individuals and then co-hybridizing the DNA to a normal metaphase chromosomal preparation. If one DNA sample has any major chromosomal deletion then the ratio of colours hybridizing to that region on the normal chromosomes will be different from the rest. This technique is particularly useful in characterizing tumour DNA

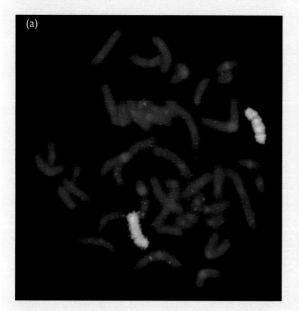 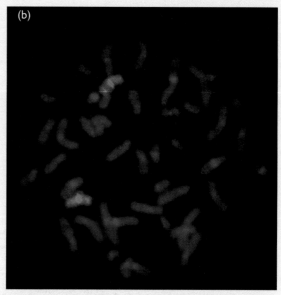

Fig. 2.9 Chromosome painting of chromosome 10 (a) and chromosome 11 (b). (Fig. (a) supplied by Dr Shelagh Boyle.)

BOX 2.17 MOLECULAR CYTOGENETICS (Cont.)

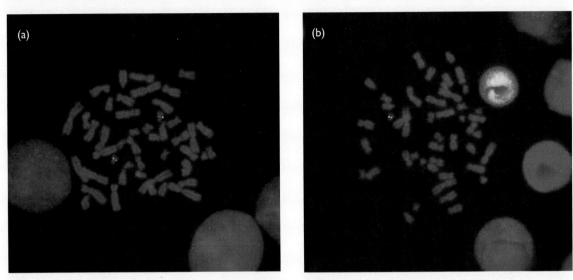

Fig. 2.10 Chromosome metaphase spreads with 22q11 specific fluorescent probe showing (a) signal on both chromosome 22s in a normal control and (b) only one signal in a patient with a microdeletion in this area.

Fig. 2.11

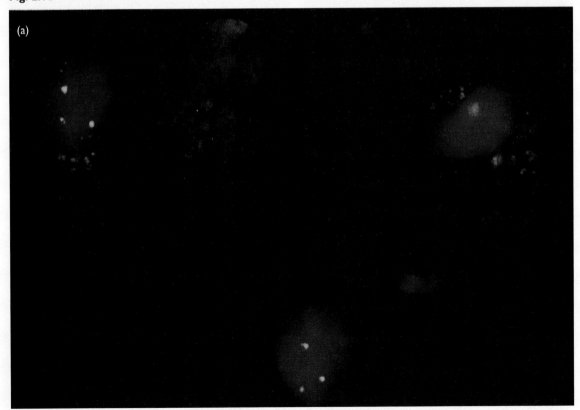

BOX 2.17 MOLECULAR CYTOGENETICS (Cont.)

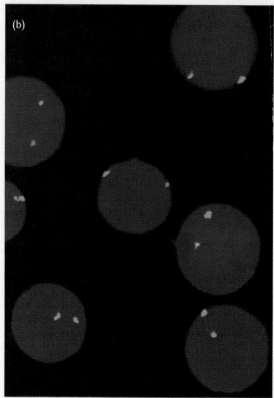

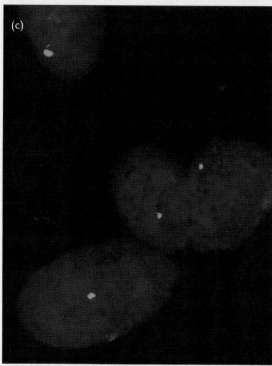

Fig. 2.11 Interphase FISH with (a) chromosome 21 specific YAC probe showing trisomy 21 in a patient with Down syndrome, (b) X chromosome probe (green) in a female patient and (c) X chromosome specific probe (green) and Y specific probe (red) in a male patient. (Figures (b) and (c) were supplied by Dr J P Warner and Mr T Johnston and figure (a) was supplied by Mrs Avril Morris.)

BOX 2.18 MICRODELETION SYNDROMES

◆ **Williams syndrome** – del(7)(q11.23), results in deletion of the elastin gene, supravalvular aortic stenosis, characteristic face and behaviour, hypercalcaemia

◆ **Langer–Giedion** – del(8)(q24.11q24.13), results in exostoses (bony lumps), unusual nose, mental handicap

◆ **WAGR syndrome** – del(11)(p13), results in Wilms tumour, aniridia, genitourinary abnormalities, mental handicap

◆ **Prader–Willi/Angelman syndrome** – del(15) (q11). These two distinct conditions may be caused by deletions in the same chromosomal region and will be discussed further in Chapter 8

◆ **Rubinstein–Taybi syndrome** – del(16)(p13.3),

causes mental handicap, long nasal columella, broad thumbs

◆ **Miller–Dieker syndrome** – del(17)(p13.3), causes lissencephaly (smooth brain)

◆ **Smith–Magenis syndrome** – del(17)(p11.2), results in behavioural problems, mental handicap

◆ **Di George syndrome** (DGS) – del(22) (q11.22), see Case 2.5

◆ **Velo-cardio-facial syndrome** – del(22) (q11.22). This is caused by a microdeletion in the same region as DGS. Cleft palate, heart defects, mental handicap and a characteristic face are common features

◆ **Azoospermia** – del(Y)(q11.23), causes male infertility

QUESTIONS (ANSWERS ON PAGE 167)

1 Human chromosomes are
a composed entirely of DNA.
b the most numerous of any species.
c normally located in the cytosol.
d present only in actively-dividing tissues.
e normally identified by Giemsa-induced banding patterns.

2 Human chromosome analysis by light microscopy
a can only be performed on peripheral blood cells.
b is easiest when chromosomes are decondensed.
c is now usually performed by a computer in ~1 h.
d can usually detect deletions $>4 \times 10^6$ base-pairs in size.
e is a useful investigation in couples with recurrent early miscarriages.

3 Trisomy of chromosome
a 21 is usually the result of an error in maternal mitosis.
b 21 is associated with increased paternal age.
c 18 is often found in apparently normal children.
d 13 occurs in 1 in 600 births.
e 21 occurs almost exclusively in women over 35 years of age.

4 If the chromosomal constitution of an individual was
a 46,XX, they would have two active X chromosomes in each cell.
b 45,X, they would usually have ambiguous external genitalia.
c 47,XXY they would be infertile.
d 47,XXX they would be infertile.
e 45,X they have a high risk of significant short stature.

5 Reciprocal translocations
a only occur between acrocentric chromosomes.
b are rarely inherited.
c rarely cause disease in carriers.
d often result in a 5% or greater risk of chromosome aneuploidy in offspring of carriers.
e may cause male infertility.

6 FISH analysis
a can be performed on uncultured cells.
b requires specialized microscopes.
c can detect small deletions in DNA ($<1 \times 10^6$).
d is used instead of light microscopy for routine chromosome analysis.
e can be used to map genes chromosomally.

7 Robertsonian translocations
a most commonly involve chromosome 13.
b involve fusion of metacentric chromosomes.
c generally result in higher reproductive risk in female carriers than male.
d are the cause of ~25% of Down syndrome.
e can result in the formation of a chromosome with two centromeres.

8 Extra structurally abnormal chromosomes (ESAC)
a containing euchromatic material are usually benign.
b often contain chromosome 15 material.
c can be identified using molecular cytogenetic techniques.
d may be associated with cat-eye syndrome.
e are never inherited.

9 Down syndrome
a may be associated with presenile dementia.
b shows marked differences in incidence between races.
c is particularly associated with atrioventricular septal defects.
d causes no predisposition to malignancy.
e critical region is on 21p.

10 Giemsa-pale bands (R-bands) on human metaphase chromosomes
a contain almost all widely expressed human genes.
b are GC-rich.
c contain tandemly repeated segments of DNA.
d are commonly involved in heteromorphisms.
e are not present on the X chromosome.

3

Molecular Genetics

LEARNING OBJECTIVES

After studying this chapter, the reader should understand:

- the physical relationship between the chromosome and the DNA it contains
- the way the genome is functionally organized
- the main structural components of a gene
- the types of mutation which underlie genetic
- disease and the technologies required to analyse them
- the meaning of allelic heterogeneity in genetic diseases and the practical limitations that this imposes on mutation screening

INTRODUCTION

In the previous chapter the structure and behaviour of chromosomes were described. A large part of the information in it could be deduced by observing the chromosomes directly under the light microscope. However, much of the complexity of human genetics, and most of the information about the way in which the genome is expressed, is only revealed by analysis of chromosomes and the DNA contained within them at a much finer, molecular, level than permitted by cytogenetics.

Chromosomes are the inherited elements through which the genetic material is transmitted, and within the chromosomes, the information-carrying component is the DNA. Therefore, although chromosomes contain many structural components other than DNA, the study of inheritance can be reduced almost entirely to the study of DNA sequences. This requires the use of molecular biological techniques, mostly developed since the 1970s, some of which are described in this book. Understanding the rules governing inheritance of genes requires knowledge of their DNA structure, and also of the relationship

between chromosomes and the DNA they contain (Fig. 3.1).

CHROMOSOMES AND DNA

Mammalian chromosomes are linear and each has two ends (telomeres). Corresponding to this shape and visible down the microscope, each chromosome contains a single linear dsDNA molecule. Although the DNA in chromosomes is packaged in complex coils along with histones and other important structural proteins, from a purely genetic point of view the chromosome can be regarded as a linear DNA molecule (though this DNA molecule would be several cm long if stretched out fully).

Chemical structure of DNA

DNA is a string of deoxyribose sugars, joined by phosphate groups between two of their carbon atoms at the positions known as 5' ("5 prime") and 3'. This sugar-phosphate chain has **direction**; at one end it has an unconnected 5' sugar group

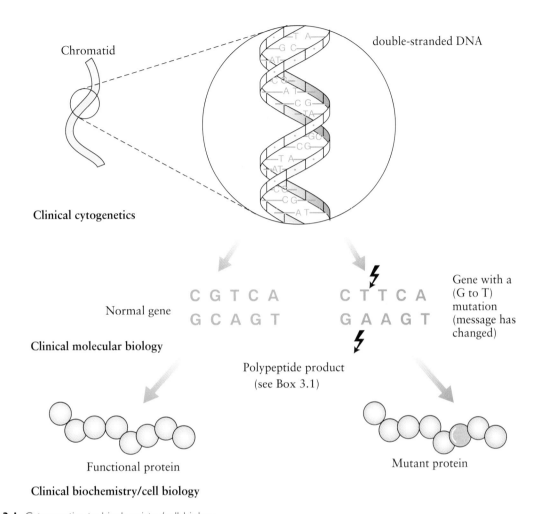

Fig. 3.1 Cytogenetics to biochemistry/cell biology.

and at the other a 3'. To the side of each sugar is attached one of four possible nucleotide bases: adenine, cytosine, guanine or thymine (A, C, G or T). The sequence of these bases is referred to as the DNA sequence, read from 5' → 3' as indicated in Fig. 3.2 by the arrow.

The DNA of all higher organisms is double-stranded. This means that two sugar-phosphate chains, running in opposite directions, are twined round each other in the well-known double-helical

(a)

(b)

Sequence: ACGT

Fig. 3.2 (a) Deoxyribose, the five-carbon sugar found in DNA. In RNA, ribose is found instead, which differs only by an extra –OH group on the 2' carbon atom. Note the position of the 5' and 3' carbon atoms where the phosphate groups are attached in DNA.
(b) The structure of a single strand of DNA. A=adenine, C=cytosine, G=guanine, T=thymine, P=phosphate.

structure deduced in the 1950s by Crick and Watson. The two strands are held together by hydrogen-bonding between their bases, according to the simple rule by which A on one strand is paired with T on the other, and C with G. Because of this base-pairing rule, the sequence of one strand can be completely predicted from that of the other, and the two strands are said to be complementary. When DNA sequences are described, only one strand is usually written; thus a sequence

5'–AACGTTCGGCCGGTAA

may be written where the actual meaning is the dsDNA sequence

5'–AACGTTCGGCCGGTAA
TTGCAAGCCGGCCATT–5'

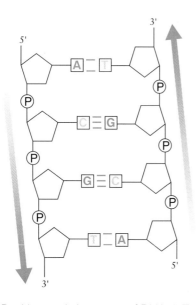

Fig. 3.3 Double-stranded structure of DNA. A:T and G:C base pairs are held together by hydrogen bonding. The two complementary strands run in opposite directions, 5' to 3'.

The double-stranded structure of DNA is shown in Fig. 3.3. At DNA replication, the strands of the double helix separate and each serves as a template for the synthesis of a new second strand. The result is two double helices in place of one (Chapter 2, Fig. 2.4).

Methylation of DNA

Although synthesized from the four nucleotides referred to above, human DNA also undergoes modifications after it is synthesized, the most important being methylation of cytosine bases. This occurs predominantly at CG dinucleotides, which are rarer than expected in mammalian DNA. CG methylation (often referred to as CpG methylation) often occurs when a gene is transcriptionally inactive. On a large scale, this also applies to the inactive X chromosome in females (Chapter 7), which is heavily methylated. Conversely, when a gene is activated, demethylation often occurs of DNA in a CpG-rich region associated with the 5' end of the gene. These CpG regions are referred to as CpG islands.

THE GENETIC CODE AND DISEASE

The functional units within DNA are called genes. Classically one gene contains the information to form one protein. Each gene is transcribed within the nucleus into an RNA copy of one strand. The RNA is processed in various ways within the nucleus (**Box 3.1**). The RNAs (known as messenger RNAs, mRNA) are exported to the cytoplasm where they act as templates for protein synthesis (translation) by the ribosome. Protein synthesis involves the addition of amino acids into chains to form proteins. Each individual amino acid is coded for in the mRNA by a three nucleotide base sequence, a codon. Since there are 64 possible codons obtainable from the four nucleotide bases, but only 20 amino acids participating in protein synthesis, most amino acids have more than one codon (**Box 3.2**). Protein synthesis starts with the initiation codon ATG (methionine) and ends with one of the three stop codons TAA, TGA or TAG.

Allelic heterogeneity in genetic disease

It is well known that any complicated piece of machinery – a computer for example – can be caused to malfunction in a variety of ways (remove CPU, mechanically damage hard drive, etc.). It is therefore not surprising that most genes can be and

BOX 3.1 GENE STRUCTURE AND TRANSCRIPTION

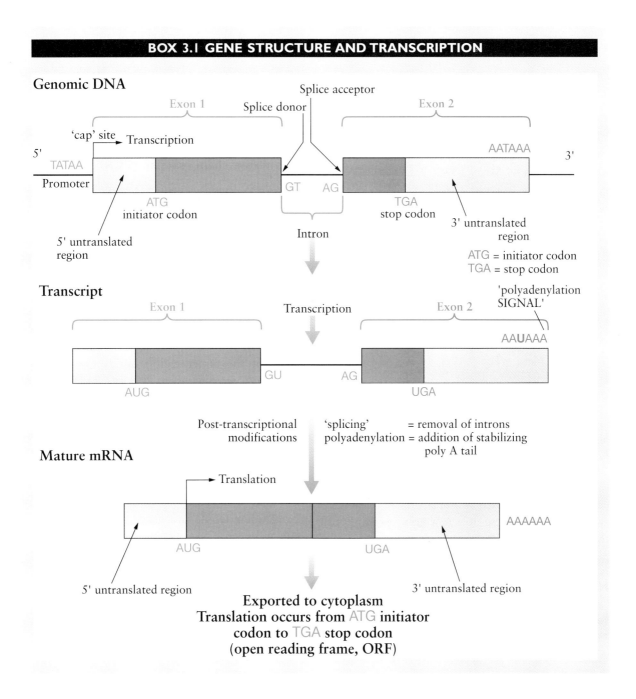

Genomic DNA

Splice acceptor

Exon 1   Splice donor   Exon 2

'cap' site   Transcription

5'   AATAAA   3'

TATAA   GT   AG

Promoter   TGA

ATG   stop codon

initiator codon

3' untranslated region

5' untranslated region   Intron   ATG = initiator codon
                                                TGA = stop codon

Transcript

'polyadenylation SIGNAL'

Exon 1   Transcription   Exon 2

AAU**A**AA

GU   AG

AUG   UGA

Post-transcriptional   'splicing'   = removal of introns
modifications   polyadenylation = addition of stabilizing
                                    poly A tail

Mature mRNA

Translation

AAAAAA

AUG   UGA

5' untranslated region   3' untranslated region

Exported to cytoplasm
Translation occurs from ATG **initiator**
codon to TGA **stop codon**
(open reading frame, ORF)

are inactivated by any one of a variety of different mutations within them (**Box 3.3**). Since each different 'variant' of a gene is called an allele, this phenomenon is known as allelic heterogeneity. The next chapter demonstrates the practical difficulties caused by allelic heterogeneity. In general, as a result of allelic heterogeneity, for most genetic diseases, particularly recessive ones (in which a gene

function is usually lost), there is no way of knowing which particular mutation within the gene has caused the disease in an individual patient. Exceptions to this general principle do exist; the sickle cell anaemia (Case 3.1) is one such. Also, for some dominantly inherited conditions where the molecular pathology does not cause a *loss* of function, but a specific *alteration* of function, only

BOX 3.2 THE GENETIC CODE

1st position (5' end) ↓	2nd position T	C	A	G	3rd position (3' end) ↓
T	Phe	Ser	Tyr	Cys	T
	Phe	Ser	Tyr	Cys	C
	Leu	Ser	STOP	STOP	A
	Leu	Ser	STOP	Trp	G
C	Leu	Pro	His	Arg	T
	Leu	Pro	His	Arg	C
	Leu	Pro	Gln	Arg	A
	Leu	Pro	Gln	Arg	G
A	Ile	Thr	Asn	Ser	T
	Ile	Thr	Asn	Ser	C
	Ile	Thr	Lys	Arg	A
	Met	Thr	Lys	Arg	G
G	Val	Ala	Asp	Gly	T
	Val	Ala	Asp	Gly	C
	Val	Ala	Glu	Gly	A
	Val	Ala	Glu	Gly	G

one or a very few mutations may be capable of causing that particular biochemical change. Achondroplasia (Case 3.2) is a good example of this.

MOLECULAR TECHNIQUES

Restriction endonucleases ('restriction enzymes')

Valuable tools for use in many areas of molecular genetics are provided by a wide variety of restriction endonucleases, which are produced by many microorganisms. These enyzmes recognize specific dsDNA sequences (often short 'palindromes' where the sequence is the same on both antiparallel strands, e.g. GGATCC or GAATTC) and then cut the DNA. Consequently, restriction enzymes allow the cleavage of DNA molecules at defined positions, which is very useful for genetic manipulation. Furthermore, since a change of a single

base-pair within the recognition site will abolish cleavage, restriction enzymes can also be used to detect variation in DNA sequence at specific sites. An application of this for mutation detection is shown in case 3.1; the use of restriction enzymes for other purposes is described in Chapter 4.

Polymerase chain reaction (PCR)

Modern molecular genetics is heavily dependent on the polymerase chain reaction (PCR), an enzymatic technique for DNA amplification, invented in 1985 by Kary Mullis, who later received the Nobel prize for chemistry for the invention. Amplification in this context means not increase in size but increase in the number of molecules of a chosen target region of DNA (**Box 3.4**). To be able to analyse the structure of a region of DNA (part of the gene of interest) by simple chemical methods, the molecules of the target region must be visible, for example by staining a gel. PCR can easily increase the number of target copies by 100 million fold in a matter of 2–3 h, in a test tube. Thus, starting for example from a small amount (about 100 ng) of hugely complex human genomic DNA, a large amount (1 μg) of a homogenous 300 base-pair target sequence can be produced. This sequence is a copy of the corresponding target region from the genomic DNA, and hence can be analysed to indicate the presence of any pathogenic mutation in the original DNA.

Electrophoresis

Electrophoresis is the most important method used to separate mixtures of DNA molecules. The phosphates in the DNA backbone make DNA strongly negatively charged. Under the influence of an electric current, therefore, DNA molecules migrate towards the positive electrode (anode). If the electrophoresis is performed in a semisolid support such as agarose or polyacrylamide gel, a 'sieving' effect causes smaller molecules to migrate faster than large ones. This allows separation and accurate size estimation of DNA fragments, such as those derived from restriction digest or from PCR. A reference lane consisting of a mixture of DNA

BOX 3.3 TYPES OF MUTATIONS

Point mutations

◆ Missense   Alters an amino acid, which can cause a change in charge, structural conformation or may affect a binding site of the protein.

◆ Nonsense   Alters an amino acid codon to a stop codon. This results in a truncated protein and therefore is likely to have a severe effect on the protein's function unless the mutation occurs very close to the end of the coding region.

Deletions

◆ Intragenic   *Out-of-frame deletion*. If the deletion involves one or more nucleotides, not a multiple of three, then the codon sequence downstream of the mutation will be disturbed. This frameshift mutation usually causes the altered reading frame to eventually contain a stop codon (TGA, TAA or TAG), so that a truncated protein is usually produced.

In-frame deletion. If the deletion involves a multiple of three nucleotides then only the corresponding amino acids will be deleted from the protein.

An analogy would be: This line can be read well

in-frame deletion: This line be read well

out-of-frame deletion: This Lnec anb er eadwell

◆ Contiguous gene syndrome
   If a deletion is very large, a number of neighbouring genes may be removed, so that the function of more than one gene is lost.

Specific targets

◆ Splice junction
   Splicing of introns requires specific, invariant sequences around the splice junctions: GT . . . and . . . AG dinucleotides begin and end the intron. Alteration in these sequences impairs or prevents correct splicing, causing aberrant mRNA to be made.

◆ Promoter / polyadenylation signals
   Alters transcription of the gene or prevents the addition of the poly (A) tail, which is essential for the stability of most mRNAs.

Trinucleotide repeats
   See Chapter 8, Box 8.1.

fragments of known sizes is run beside the test samples. After electrophoresis, the DNA is usually visualized by staining the gel with a fluorescent dye, ethidium bromide, which binds to DNA. Alternative methods are also sometimes used, such as radioactively labelling the DNA and then detecting it by exposing the gel to X-ray film. **Southern blotting** A method for detecting specific sequences within a complex DNA mixture (**Box 3.5**).

BOX 3.4 POLYMERASE CHAIN REACTION TECHNIQUE

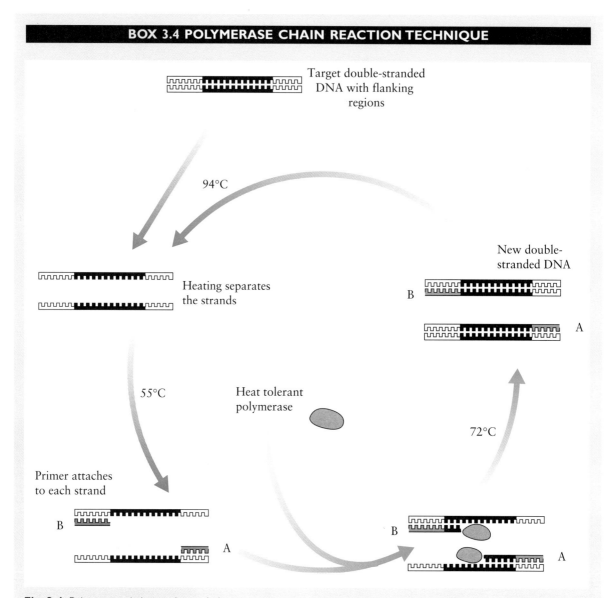

Fig. 3.4 Polymerase chain reaction technique.

The initial double-stranded template DNA is separated into strands ('denatured') at 94°C and then cooled back to 55°C to allow two short synthetic oligonucleotides to anneal, one to each strand. These serve as primers to define the start of DNA synthesis (copying of template strands) at 72°C by a thermostable DNA polymerase. After this first round (usually taking about 3 min), the temperature cycle is repeated about 30 times, giving an initially exponential increase in the number of copies of the target region between the two primers. Note that in the second and subsequent rounds, the polymerase terminates DNA synthesis at the end of a template strand corresponding to the position of the primer in the previous round. Two of the four new strands made are thus of defined length. After a few more rounds of synthesis, these fixed-length products are the predominant species in the reaction.

BOX 3.5 SOUTHERN BLOTTING

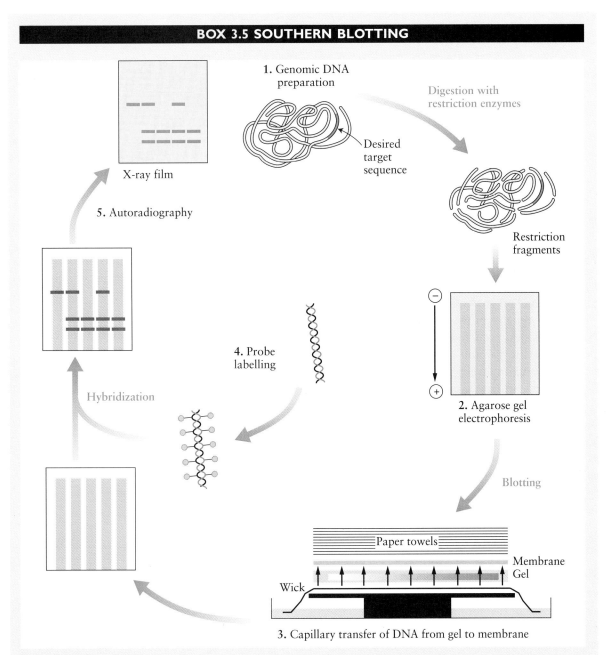

Fig. 3.5 Southern blotting.

(1) The genomic DNA is digested by restriction enzymes into fragments of DNA. The two copies of a gene may be cut into fragments of differing lengths. (2) These fragments are then separated out by gel electrophoresis, the larger fragments moving least and remaining at the top of the gel. (3) The DNA is then transferred from the gel to a membrane by capillary action. The DNA is then fixed onto the membrane by UV irradiation..(4) DNA probes (small DNA fragments, complementary in sequence to the gene under investigation) are labelled with a radioactive tag and allowed to bind to the DNA on the membrane. (5) The membrane is then exposed to radiation-sensitive film and the DNA fragments to which the probe has bound form a band on the film. As the two copies (alleles) of a gene generate fragments of different sizes, different banding patterns may be seen in each individual seen in each individual.

CASE 3.1
Sickle cell anaemia

Family tree

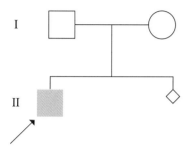

Presenting complaint

Leonard and Sarah were referred for advice during her second pregnancy. Their first child, Robbie (II-1), had been diagnosed at age 18 months as suffering from sickle cell anaemia. He had originally presented with painful swellings of his fingers (dactylitis) and on investigation had been found to have a hypochromic anaemia with characteristic sickle-shaped deformed red blood cells on the blood film. The diagnosis was confirmed by haemoglobin electrophoresis, which showed an abnormally migrating haemoglobin S band in place of the usual haemoglobin A band. Leonard and Sarah were concerned about this pregnancy also being affected.

What is sickle cell disease?

Sickle cell disease is an autosomal recessive disorder in which abnormal haemoglobin (HbS) is synthesized in place of the normal haemoglobin A (HbA). Normal haemoglobin A has the tetrameric structure $\alpha_2\beta_2$. In the common form of sickle cell anaemia, a glutamate (Glu) to valine (Val) substitution at position 6 of the β globin gene causes the abnormal properties of the HbS. HbS has a tendency to form aggregates under conditions of low pH or hypoxia, deforming the red cells which then themselves aggregate and occlude microvasculature. This sets up a vicious cycle of hypoxic damage to tissues; sickle cell disease is characterized by repeated painful occlusive episodes, particularly affecting bones, by lung infarction and infection, by cerebrovascular accidents, by haemolytic anaemia, and by susceptibility to infection (especially with pneumococcus, due to splenic infarction).

What genetic advice can be offered?

As an autosomal recessive condition, the recurrence risk for sickle anaemia is 1 in 4. Leonard and Sarah decide they wish prenatal diagnosis in the current pregnancy. This cannot easily be performed by analysis of the abnormal protein product, since fetal red blood cells would be needed, and these contain very little HbA or HbS until very late in pregnancy. (The fetus makes its own forms of embryonic and fetal haemoglobin, which do not contain the β chain.) Prenatal diagnosis must therefore be by DNA analysis.

How is the DNA sample analysed for the presence of the known mutation?

Sickle cell anaemia results from a β^6 glutamate to valine amino acid change, due to a single base mutation shown in Fig. 3.6.

The DNA sequence around codon 6 of the β globin gene is shown, along with the encoded amino-acids underneath. A useful feature of the

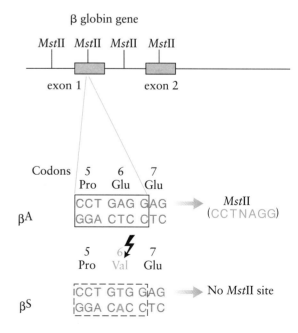

Fig. 3.6 Single-base mutation in the β globin gene.

BOX 3.6 EXAMPLE OF HOW A MUTATION CAN BE TYPED BY PCR

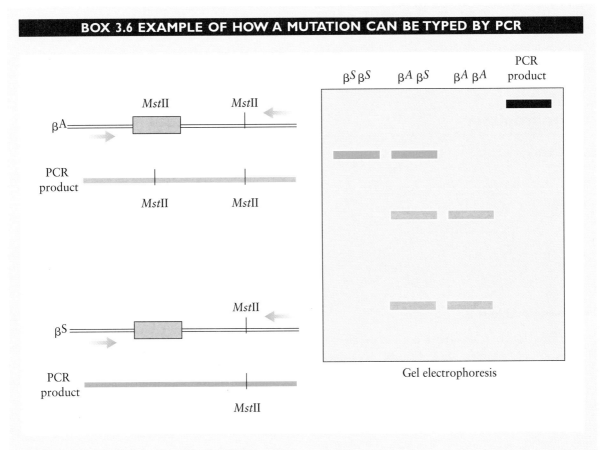

Fig. 3.7 Analysis of sickle cell mutation by PCR.

In Fig. 3.7 the PCR product (thick line) is defined by the position of the two **primers** (arrows) flanking *Mst*II sites in the **genomic** DNA (thin double lines). One of these *Mst*II sites is the site of the sickle cell mutation, the other serves as a control for complete digestion of the PCR product. The resulting electrophoretic patterns are shown to the right. A normal allele (A) cuts at both *Mst*II sites, while a sickle allele (S) cuts at the right-hand site only. Cleavage at the right-hand site confirms that the failure of the codon 6 site to cleave is not due to a technical problem with the restriction digest.

DNA sequence here is that it contains the recognition sequence for the restriction enzyme *Mst*II, as shown boxed. This recognition sequence is abolished by the A to T change causing sickle cell disease. This fact can be easily used to test a PCR product containing the mutation site for the presence or absence of the *Mst*II site, and hence the normal or mutated sequence (**Box 3.6**).

For Leonard and Sarah, as they presented only at 15 weeks' gestation, the prenatal diagnosis was performed by amniocentesis rather than chorionic villus sampling (see Chapter 6). Since PCR requires only very small amounts of DNA, enough material was obtained directly from the amniotic cell pellet, without the need to culture it, giving a rapid result within 24 h. The fetus was found to be heterozygous for the mutation, and hence predicted to be a carrier, that is to have sickle cell trait.

What effect does sickle cell trait have on the fetus?

As is the rule for autosomal recessive diseases,

sickle cell carriers are usually asymptomatic. However, they are at risk of haemolysis and other problems under hypoxic stress. This is likely to be most important during anaesthesia.

CASE 3.2
Achondroplasia

Family tree

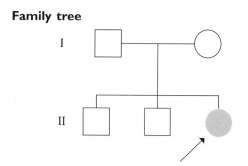

Presenting problem

Angela was born at term after a normal pregnancy. Her father and mother, aged 47 and 43 respectively, already had two healthy teenage children, and the present pregnancy had been unintended but not unwelcome. At delivery, it was immediately noted that Angela's arms and legs were short, and a paediatric opinion was sought. On examination, there was marked shortening of the proximal segments of all four limbs. She had a prominent forehead and depressed nasal bridge. Her hands were broad, with a gap between the middle and third fingers giving a three-pronged 'trident' appearance. A clinical diagnosis of achondroplasia was made in Angela.

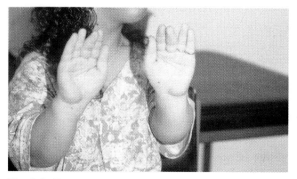

Fig. 3.8 Photograph of trident hand associated with achrondoplasia in a young adult.

What is achondroplasia?

Achondroplasia is one of the commoner short-limbed skeletal dysplasias, with a frequency estimated variously at 1 in 10 000 to 1 in 50 000. It is an autosomal dominant condition, with a 50% risk for affected individuals to have affected offspring. Short stature is the main problem in achondroplasia, but there is also an increased risk of sudden infant death due to cervical spinal cord compression. Women with achondroplasia usually require Caesarian section at the end of pregnancy because of their small pelvic dimensions.

How can the diagnosis be confirmed?

Achondroplasia is due to the specific mutation glycine to arginine at amino acid 380 (G380R) within the fibroblast growth factor receptor type 3 (*FGFR3*) gene on chromosome 4p16.3. About 80% of these are new mutations since both parents (as in this case) are normal in height (and do not carry the mutation). There is a slightly increased average paternal age in these new mutation cases, suggesting an increased risk of a new mutation in spermatogenesis as the father gets older. Since two affected parents marry more frequently than one would expect from the population frequency, the birth of a child homozygous for the G380R mutation is an occasional occurrence. Unfortunately, such homozygous babies have an extreme short-limbed lethal asphyxiating skeletal dysplasia. First trimester prenatal diagnosis for such couples is possible by DNA analysis. As in the case of sickle cell anaemia, this test for a single point mutation requires a single PCR and one or two restriction enzyme digests for its demonstration.

What was the result of the mutation analysis in Angela?

The clinical suspicion of achondroplasia was in this case confirmed by the DNA test. DNA from a blood sample was analysed for the presence of the mutation (G380R) in the *FGFR3* gene. The mutation was found in heterozygous state. After this, further confirmation of the diagnosis is not

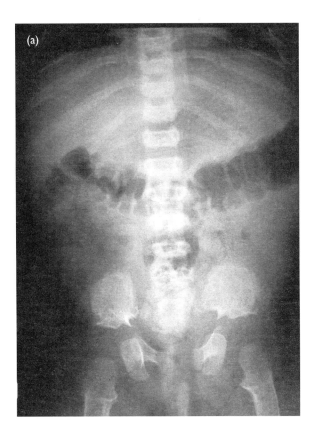 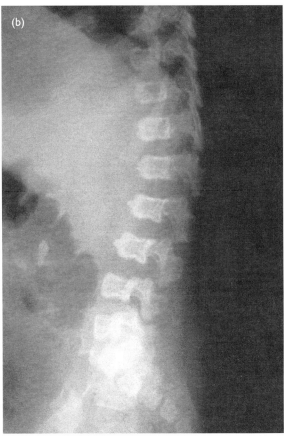

Fig. 3.9 Typical radiological features of achondroplasia: square iliac wings, narrow sacrosciatic notch ('champagne glass' outline to pelvic shadow), interpedicular distance progressively narrowing from L1–5 vertebrae (a); lumbar lordosis, posterior scalloping and anterior breaking of vertebrae (b).

required. However, it is more usual to make an unequivocal diagnosis of achondroplasia from X-ray examination (Fig. 3.9).

It should be noted that the ability to confirm or rule out a suspected clinical diagnosis by a single DNA test, as in achondroplasia, is unusual. Allelic heterogeneity sees to it that for most genetic disease, such a single DNA test does not exist.

FURTHER READING

Strachan T, Read A (1996) *Human Molecular Genetics*. BIOS Scientific Publishers Ltd, Oxford.

QUESTIONS (ANSWERS ON PAGE 168)

1 Which of the following are features of the structure of human DNA?

a It contains only one sugar (deoxyribose).

b It has the same basic chemical structure as bacterial DNA.

c The four types of base are held together in strands by phosphate groups.

d Guanine base-pairs with cytosine and adenine with uracil.

e The two strands of double-stranded DNA run in opposite directions.

2 The following are consequences of the double-stranded structure of DNA

a The sequence of one strand can be predicted from the sequence of the other.

b DNA sequences are all palindromic.

c The two strands must be separated to allow replication to take place.

d Either strand can encode a gene.

e On any one chromosome, all the genes are transcribed from the same strand.

3 The following are true of restriction endonucleases

a They can be isolated from various mammalian species.

b Each restriction endonuclease has a unique sequence specificity.

c Most restriction enzymes will only cut double-stranded DNA.

d Some restriction enzymes can cut more than one recognition sequence.

e Some restriction enzymes are sensitive to methylation of DNA.

4 DNA and chromosomes

a Mammalian chromosomes are huge supercoiled circles of double-stranded DNA.

b Centromeres of mammalian chromosomes contain a great deal of repetitive DNA.

c At mitosis, a human cell contains four copies of the DNA sequence comprising each gene.

d At mitosis, the two strands of the double-stranded DNA separate from each other into different daughter cells.

e All the DNA in a cell is in the nucleus.

5 The polymerase chain reaction

a depends on the use of an enzyme, originally isolated from a bacterium found in hot springs.

b allows the scientist to analyse a chosen segment of genomic DNA simply by specifying the sequences of the oligonucleotide primers.

c has the ability to analyse the DNA of a single cell.

d can be used for forensic purposes.

e can be used for the analysis of RNA.

6 Mutations

a Some diseases always result from the same mutation.

b Most diseases do not always result from the same mutation.

c Some diseases may result either from point mutations or from deletions.

d New mutations usually occur as a result of exposure of a parent to radiation or to DNA-damaging chemicals or drugs.

e It is always necessary to sequence the DNA of a patient in order to determine the presence of a mutation.

7 Splicing

   a The first two and last two bases of an exon are the almost invariant GT and AG splice signals.

   b Some genes can encode more than one protein.

   c All human genes have introns.

   d Splicing occurs in the cytoplasm after export of the mRNA precursor from the nucleus.

   e All exons encode an exact (whole) number of amino acids.

8 Genes

   a There are about 80 000 human genes.

   b Many genes belong to families of related genes.

   c Some genes do not encode proteins.

   d Structures of human genes do not show any similarity to those of bacteria.

   e Human genes can have up to 10 exons.

4

The Use and Limitations
of Genetic Linkage

LEARNING OBJECTIVES

After studying this chapter, the reader should understand:

- the main types of polymorphism and the ways in which they can be analysed
- how polymorphisms can be used to follow disease genes through families

- the limitations associated with diagnosis by linkage
- the meaning and significance of locus hetero-geneity

INTRODUCTION

The previous chapter illustrated some of the types of genetic pathology that can underlie human diseases. If a comprehensive catalogue of all possible mutations existed, together with the ability to screen patients' DNA for all these pathogenic changes, then genetic diagnosis could be reduced entirely to the simple business of testing for mutations. Unfortunately, this goal has not yet been reached and less direct methods, based on the ability to track disease-causing genes through families, are still a mainstay of diagnosis. This chapter illustrates the problems encountered and ways in which they can be solved. To understand this chapter, the reader should be thoroughly familiar with the chromosomal events in meiosis, with the structure of human DNA, and with the relationship between the cytogenetically visible chromosome and the DNA which it contains (see Chapters 2 and 3).

CASE 4.1

Cystic fibrosis with unknown mutation

Family tree

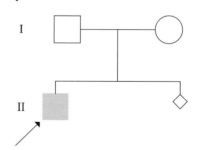

Presenting problem

Robert (II-1), aged 2½ years, has recently been investigated for failure to gain weight and repeated chest infections. On the basis of a sweat test, which showed an elevated chloride concentration, he has just been diagnosed as having cystic fibrosis. His mother, Brenda (I-2), has been referred for genetic advice at 14 weeks' gestation in her second pregnancy. She and her husband Eric have been told that the current pregnancy has a 1 in 4 chance of resulting in another child with cystic fibrosis. Though undecided as to their course of action, they have requested advice about the possibility of prenatal diagnosis.

What is cystic fibrosis?

Cystic fibrosis (CF) results from defects in the function of the cystic fibrosis transmembrane conductance regulator (CFTR), a membrane chloride channel which regulates the electrolyte composition of exocrine secretions. The resulting raised concentration of sodium and chloride in sweat forms the basis for the diagnostic sweat test, in which a sample of sweat from the child's skin is collected on a filter paper patch and the electrolyte concentrations measured.

The *CF* gene is on chromosome 7q, and since CF is an autosomal recessive disease, both copies of the gene are defective in patients with the disease. In Northern Europe, one mutation, ΔF508, is found within the majority of defective *CF* genes in patients. This mutation, which accounts for 75% of defective *CF* genes, is a three nucleotide deletion resulting in a single amino acid (phenylalanine residue 508) being missing from the CFTR protein. This deletion can be detected by PCR. The proportion of CF patients with two copies of the ΔF508 mutation is $(0.75)^2 \approx 0.5$; in other words, about half of CF patients are ΔF508 homozygotes.

What did ΔF508 mutation testing show in this family?

As Robert is clinically affected and has an abnormal sweat test, he must have a mutation in both his CFTR genes. However, investigation of the family showed that Robert was heterozygous for the ΔF508 mutation, his father Eric was also heterozygous for ΔF508, but Brenda his mother did not have the ΔF508 mutation. Since the diagnosis was not in doubt, this implied that Robert's other *CF* gene (inherited from his mother) was defective

because of the presence of a different mutation (Fig. 4.1). Unfortunately, the mutations which account for the remaining 25% of defective *CF* genes are extremely heterogeneous. Several hundred different mutations have been described, many only ever seen in one family. In a diagnostic situation, particularly when time is short, it is not feasible to test for each individual mutation since each mutation needs a separate assay to be designed for its detection.

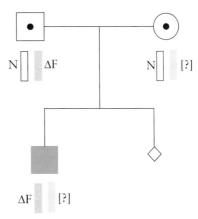

Fig. 4.1 The genetic situation deduced from analysis of the ΔF508 mutation in the CF family. The four parental copies of chromosome 7 are shown, with the two carrying the ΔF508 and unknown ([?]) mutations in dark and light shading, respectively. Both parents must have a normal (N) *CF* gene in addition to the mutated one, since they are both unaffected with the disease.

Can prenatal testing still be offered to Brenda and Eric?

Prenatal diagnosis for cystic fibrosis can only be performed by DNA analysis, since the CFTR protein is not expressed in amniocytes or chorionic villus tissue. The fetus could be tested for the ΔF508 mutation, but without knowing which maternal chromosome 7 the fetus had inherited, the presence of ΔF508 cannot distinguish between the carrier state and the affected state. What is needed is some way to distinguish between Brenda's two *CF* genes in order to determine whether the fetus had the same maternal *CF* gene as the affected boy Robert (shaded), or the opposite one (white). In the latter case, an unaffected outcome could be predicted, even if the fetus had inherited ΔF508 from the father. This is illustrated in Fig. 4.2. Each copy of chromosome 7 (or more precisely, the region of that chromosome around the *CF* gene) in the family has been 'labelled' or 'marked' with a letter *a–d* (any other, arbitrary, numerical or alphabetical labels could be used).

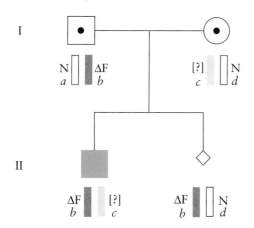

Fig. 4.2 DNA marker distinguish between parental chromosomes so that a chromosome with a mutation can be tracked through a family.

Note how this new data is interpreted. Robert must have inherited an unidentified mutation ([?]) from his mother Brenda. The *c*-labelled chromosome is the one which has been passed to Robert from his mother. Therefore, in Brenda it is *c* which marks the chromosome carrying the unknown mutation, and *d* which marks her normal chromosome.

What was the result of the prenatal diagnosis?

Brenda and Eric opted to have prenatal diagnosis in the current pregnancy, the result of which is also shown (Fig. 4.2). Amniocentesis performed at 16 weeks' gestation was used to obtain cells, from which enough DNA can be prepared to allow rapid PCR-based testing for both the known mutation ΔF508 and the 'labels' or 'markers' *a–d* for the copies of chromosome 7. The fetus has inherited the *d* chromosome from Brenda, and is therefore predicted to be an unaffected CF carrier.

What is the real nature of 'markers'?

Many of the inherited differences between individuals are obvious. Phenotypic traits such as pigmentation and height are partly genetically determined and show variation between individuals. The genes determining these features may thus be said to be polymorphic (occurring as more than one normal variant). However, there is much more polymorphic variation in DNA than is obvious phenotypically. This is fortunate, as it allows geneticists to distinguish between the two homologous copies of any chromosome (or chromosomal region) which an individual has inherited, one from each parent. If the two copies of a gene or DNA segment possessed by an individual are distinguishable, they are known as different alleles of that gene.

On average, the DNA sequence of any two haploid genomes derived from unrelated parents will differ about every 300 nucleotides; unrelated humans are about 99.7% identical to each other. The two commonest types of polymorphism are single nucleotide changes (**Box 4.1**) and variable number tandem repeats (VNTRs) (**Box 4.2**).

To be useful in diagnosis, a polymorphism simply has to allow discrimination between the two copies of the chromosomal region within which it lies; it does not have to be involved in any way in *causing* the genetic disease in question. Note in Fig. 4.2 that vital information required to perform the prenatal diagnosis comes from the previous affected child, Robert. If he had died (and no DNA or tissue had been stored), it would not have been possible to determine which maternal allele (*c* or *d*) marked Brenda's normal and which her mutated gene. Storage of DNA from individuals affected with genetic diseases, even if no tests are planned at the time of sampling, can allow important questions to be answered many years later.

What are the limitations of diagnosis by genetic linkage?

● Lack of key family members required for interpretation of the data may prevent a test from being performed. Linkage testing is a procedure which requires analysis of families, and can never be applied to isolated individuals, or apparently sporadic cases of a disease. Undisclosed non-paternity may also render the family analysis totally inaccurate.

BOX 4.1 SINGLE NUCLEOTIDE CHANGES – RFLPS

A single nucleotide change (such as a substitution of T for C) often results in the gain or loss of a recognition site for one particular restriction enzyme. These changes may therefore be detected as (and loosely referred to as) restriction fragment length polymorphisms or RFLPs. Unlike the pathogenic mutation in sickle cell anaemia, loss or gain of these restriction enzyme recognition sites does not cause disease. They reflect normal DNA variation. However, they are detected by similar techniques to those used in detection of the sickle cell mutation, namely PCR (Chapter 3, Case 3.1) or Southern blotting (Chapter 3, Fig. 3.5).

The limitation of this type of polymorphism is that since the enzyme restriction site is either present or absent, there are only two distinguishable alleles (arbitrarily referred to here as a and b). Thus there are only three possible genotypes which any individual can have (aa, bb, or ab). When using an RFLP of this kind, there is therefore a good chance that any two chromosomes being compared will both have the same allele (i.e. that the individual will be homozygous aa or bb). The polymorphism is then not informative since the allelic copies cannot be distinguished. All these genotypes, and their appearance if inherited within a family, are shown in Fig. 4.3.

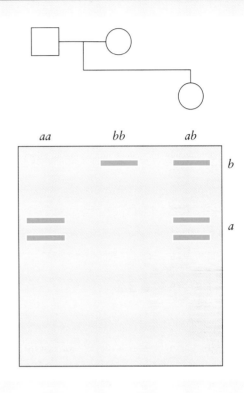

Fig. 4.3 The a allele produced due to the presence of a restriction site cutting the PCR product into two small fragments, the b allele due to absence of the restriction site remains as one large fragment. This test is uninformative as it is not possible to distinguish between the two alleles in either parent.

- Linkage cannot be used to confirm a doubtful diagnosis. Unlike direct mutation analysis, the actual mutation causing the disease is never observed in a linkage-based test, and so the diagnosis of the disease in question must be secure on other grounds *before* a linkage can be used predictively. The most important fact to bear in mind concerning the use of polymorphisms to analyse families with inherited diseases is that they are normal variants, not pathological ones
- Genetic recombination (**Box 4.3**) occurs normally and can cause the polymorphism used as a marker and the disease gene being tracked to part company. The closer the polymorphism is to the gene being tracked, the lower the risk that recombination will occur.

BOX 4.2 VNTR POLYMORPHISMS

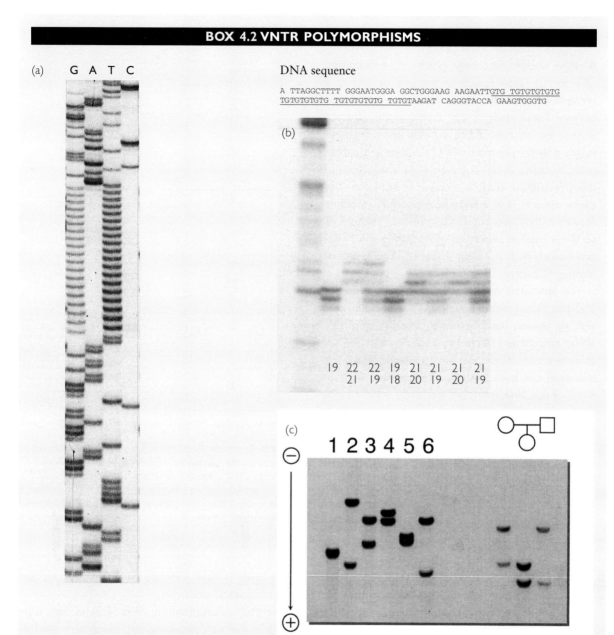

(a) G A T C

DNA sequence

A TTAGGCTTTT GGGAATGGGA GGCTGGGAAG AAGAATTGTG TGTGTGTGTG
TGTGTGTGTG TGTGTGTGTG TGTGTAAGAT CAGGGTACCA GAAGTGGGTG

(b)

19 22 22 19 21 21 21 21
21 19 18 20 19 20 19

(c) 1 2 3 4 5 6

Fig. 4.4 (a) A DNA sequencing gel derived from part of the F8VWF (von Willebrand factor) gene, showing the presence of a CA repeat. The sequence is read from the bottom up, by scoring the presence of a band in each of the four lanes, A, C, G and T; the interpretation is to the left. Because the sequence flanking the CA repeat is unique and non-redundant, PCR primers can be designed to anneal specifically to these flanking sequences, allowing amplification of the repeat for estimating its size.
(b) Results of PCR amplification of the repeat shown in (a), in a set of unrelated individuals. Four different alleles are present in this sample. Although there are shadow bands resulting from imperfections of the PCR amplification, with practice interpretation of the alleles by the position of the most intense band is easy (number of CA repeats is indicated below each lane).
(c) Southern blot showing a highly informative VNTR polymorphism locus (D7S21) with multiple alleles. Each lane contains DNA from one individual and shows two distinguishable bands representing the two allelic copies of the locus (which lies in chromosome 7p22). The arrow shows the direction of electrophoresis; larger DNA fragments migrate more slowly and hence are nearer the top of the gel. The use of this polymorphism to determine which parental chromosomes have been inherited by a child is seen in the last three lanes on the right.

BOX 4.2 VNTR POLYMORPHISMS (Cont.)

Scattered around the genome are many simple tandemly repeated DNA sequences such as CACA-CACACACACA . . . These often show *variation* in the *number* of repeat units; hence the name variable number tandem repeats (VNTRs). There may be several alleles of such a polymorphism due to differing numbers of repeats, greatly improving the chances that any individual will be heterozygous. These CA repeat polymorphisms are the most widely used for linkage studies. They are readily typed by PCR, and are so numerous that there is an excellent chance of finding one within or very close to any gene. The alleles are usually arbitrarily numbered in order of size.

Figure 4.4a shows a DNA sequencing gel with the sequence surrounding a typical CA repeat. The repetitive nature of the CA repeat itself is obvious. PCR primers (Chapter 2) are designed against the unique flanking sequence, as shown. The size of the PCR product, estimated by gel electrophoresis, then allows determination of the number of CA repeat units, as shown in Fig. 4.4b.

Like other types of DNA sequence variation, the alleles of a VNTR are passed on (with equal 50% probabilities) to an individual's offspring. Their inheritance can thus be simply observed within families, and used to follow the transmission of the chromosomal segment within which they are situated. In Fig. 4.4c, the left-hand part of the panel shows a set of unrelated individuals, typed in this case by Southern blotting, for a highly polymorphic VNTR sequence. All these individuals have two distinguishable alleles. In the right-hand part of the panel, a child and its parents are shown. Transmission of one of the two alleles from each parent to the child can clearly be seen.

BOX 4.3 GENETIC RECOMBINATION

During prophase of the first meiotic division, the two homologous copies of each chromosome align and pair up. Having previously replicated its DNA, each chromosome is already composed of an

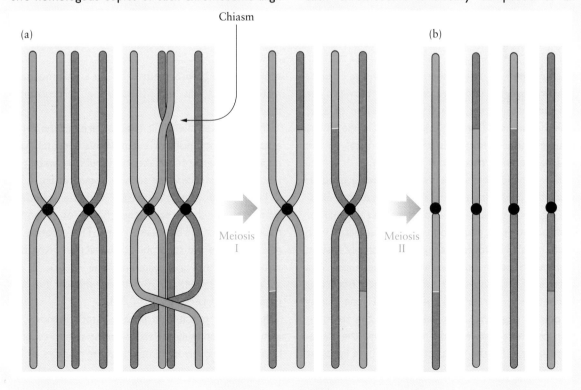

(a)

Chiasm

Meiosis I

(b)

Meiosis II

BOX 4.3 GENETIC RECOMBINATION (Cont.)

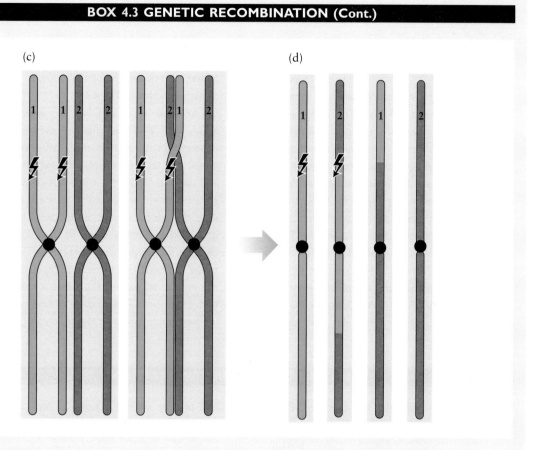

(c)　　　　　　　　　　　　　　(d)

Fig. 4.5 (a, b) Crossing over during pairing. (c, d) Reversal of phase between marker and mutation due to recombination.

identical pair of sister chromatids. During pairing crossing over, or exchange of material between the homologues, occurs at a limited number of sites called chiasmata (Fig. 4.5a). As a result, none of the resulting four chromatids will be identical to the original parental chromatids (Fig. 4.5b).

If a polymorphic DNA marker is being used to track the inheritance of an unknown mutation causing a genetic disease, it is important that the marker and the mutation in question remain associated with each other. However, if they are physically distant from each other on the chromosome, there is a chance of a crossover or recombination occurring between the marker and the mutated gene during a meiosis (Fig. 4.5c). This will reverse the relationship or phase between the marker and the mutation. In Fig. 4.5d, the mutation (shown by a lightning

strike) which before meiosis lay on a chromosome marked by *1* has ended up on a chromosome marked by *2*.

If the marker allele *1* is used to predict the presence of the mutation, for example in a prenatal diagnosis, the diagnostic prediction would be wrong in the event of a crossover such as shown in Fig. 4.5c, d. The further apart the marker and the unknown mutation are, the greater the chance of recombination occurring between them. This chance is referred to as the recombination fraction, given the symbol θ. It has a maximum value of 0.5. To be acceptable diagnostically, θ between marker and disease must be very small (<0.01).

It is never possible in linkage-based diagnosis to eliminate completely the risk of error due to recombination. Obviously it is important for markers to be

BOX 4.3 GENETIC RECOMBINATION (Cont.)

as close as possible to the gene involved in the disease. However, it is fortunately often possible to detect whether a recombination event has occurred. This is done by analysing *two* polymorphic markers, chosen such that they are on opposite sides of the gene of interest. These are known as flanking markers. The principle is shown in Fig. 4.6, using two markers A (alleles *1, 2*) and B (alleles *1, 2*). If a recom-

bination occurs, the recombinant gametes are now identifiable because, instead of the expected combinations of markers (*A1,B1* or *A2,B2*), new combinations (*A1,B2* or *A2,B1*) will be seen. This will alert the geneticist to the fact that a recombination has occurred between the markers A and B. Only if inheritance of the expected combinations *A1,B1* or *A2,B2* is seen will the linkage-based diagnosis be secure.

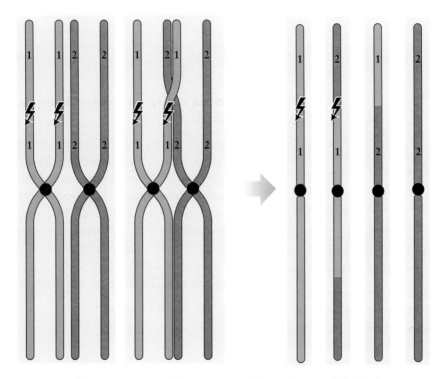

Fig. 4.6 Analysis of two flanking markers.

CASE 4.2
Carrier testing for haemophilia

Family tree

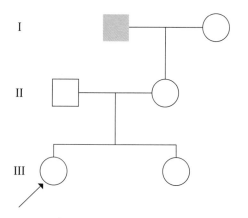

Presenting problem

Sarah (III-1) has recently married. She requests genetic advice on her risk of being a carrier of haemophilia. Her maternal grandfather (I-1) has mild haemophilia (factor VIII level ≈5% of normal levels), as a result of which he needed clotting factor VIII replacement during recent surgery.

What information of use to Sarah can be deduced from the pedigree structure *alone*?

Haemophilia A (factor VIII deficiency) is an X-linked recessive disease. Sarah's mother II-2 is therefore an *obligate carrier* of haemophilia; as the daughter of an affected male, she must carry the (undefined) factor VIII gene (*F8C*) mutation on the X chromosome which she has inherited from her father. Sarah and her sister Julia (III-2) are therefore each at 50% risk of being haemophilia carriers.

How can DNA testing by linkage resolve Sarah's carrier status?

A linkage study is undertaken using a CA repeat polymorphism which lies within intron 13 of the large *F8C* gene (an intragenic polymorphism, allowing highly accurate linkage diagnosis because of the extremely low risk of recombination between polymorphism and mutation). In the obligate carrier II-2, the *d* allele marks the abnormal *F8C* gene; the

c has come from the unaffected grandmother I-2. Note that II-1 also bears a *d* allele on his X chromosome (Fig. 4.7). *This in no way implies that he may have haemophilia!* He is an unrelated individual, whose X chromosome simply happens by chance to have the same variant of the polymorphism on it. This allele might be present on a sizeable proportion (say 20%) of X chromosomes in the general population. Polymorphisms can thus be used for following the transmission of a gene *within* a family (as from II-2 to III-1), but not, in general, for making any deductions about the status of unrelated or isolated individuals.

From Fig. 4.7, Sarah is predicted to be a carrier, since she has inherited the *d* allele which marks the *F8C* mutation in her mother.

What errors can arise in interpreting linkage data?

Sarah's sister Julia (III-2) is predicted to be a non-carrier, since she appears to have inherited the maternal *c* allele. In this case, though, there is a caveat. Julia appears to have inherited the *d* allele from her father, and hence the *c* must derive from her mother. This reasoning, however, depends on the *paternity* being correct. If Julia's biological father were unknown or in doubt, it would not be possible to be sure of her own carrier status.

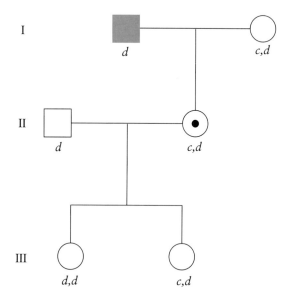

Fig. 4.7 Linkage study using an intragenic polymorphism.

Indeed, if her biological father actually had a *c* allele, the conclusion regarding her carrier status would be reversed. Thus, non-paternity can lead to false deductions in linkage-based testing, a fact which has to be borne in mind by the geneticist.

CASE 4.3
Locus heterogeneity

Family tree

Presenting problem

Amanda (III-4) was referred to the genetics clinic requesting advice about the possibility of prenatal testing for polycystic kidney disease. Several members of her family were affected and though she herself was asymptomatic, renal ultrasound scanning (see Chapter 6) had shown that both she and her older brother were in fact affected.

What is polycystic kidney disease?

Autosomal dominant polycystic kidney disease (APKD) is one of the commonest single gene disorders. Like many dominantly inherited diseases, it is a progressive condition with a variable age of clinical onset, often in middle or later life. Affected individuals develop multiple cysts in both kidneys, which progressively enlarge and may eventually destroy renal function. Early in life, the kidneys may appear normal even on ultrasound examination. APKD is thus a good example of a disease for which the penetrance is age-dependent. In addition to renal failure, APKD patients have an increased risk of subarachnoid haemorrhage due to the occurrence of intracranial berry aneurysms. Prenatal diagnosis is infrequently requested in APKD families, presumably because the disease is treatable, albeit in its end-stage only by transplantation or dialysis.

How would genetic analysis proceed in this case?

Molecular studies of the large polycystic kidney disease gene on chromosome 16p have shown that the mutations are very heterogeneous, so that routinely linkage is the only practical approach to genetic testing. Analysis of a VNTR polymorphism known to be closely linked to the *APKD* gene is shown in Fig. 4.8 (four alleles, *a–d*).

As expected, Amanda and her brother (III-3) have the same genotype *a,c*. An affected cousin III-1, however, has a different genotype, *d,d*. Conceivably such a discrepancy could be due to recombination between the VNTR marker and the disease gene, but further analysis of the family

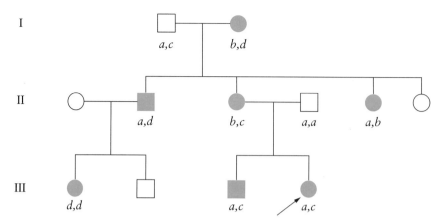

Fig. 4.8 Analysis of a VNTR polymorphism closely linked to the *APKD* gene.

shows that this is unlikely to be the case. Amanda's affected mother (II-3) inherited her mutation from her own mother, along with a *b* allele of the polymorphism. Yet, she has passed *c* to both her own affected children; both would therefore have to be recombinants to explain this result. Furthermore, Amanda's affected uncle (II-2) has inherited *d* from his affected mother (I-2), rather than the *b* inherited by his two affected sisters II-3 and II-5. At least one more recombination would therefore be needed to explain the results. The number of apparent crossovers between disease and marker in this family is so great as to call into question the prior assumption of linkage between marker and disease. Since the marker VNTR used is known to be located at 16p13, such a suggestion implies that the gene causing the polycystic kidney disease in this family may in fact not be in this chromosomal region, as originally assumed.

What is the genetic explanation?

It is known that although 95% of APKD result from mutations of the gene on chromosome 16p13, a minority of families have a clinically similar disorder, also inherited as an autosomal dominant, but in which a different gene is at fault (on chromosome 4q). This situation is known as genetic heterogeneity or locus heterogeneity. Mutation of either gene may cause APKD, and there is no way to be certain which locus is involved. This creates a serious difficulty for the use of linkage in a diagnostic setting. If it is not certain which gene is at fault, then the correct set of polymorphic markers, close to that gene, cannot be selected for following the gene through the family. A linkage study of itself, of course, gives no absolute confirmation of which locus is involved in the disease. If the family is large enough, co-segregation of the marker and the disease through generations may be seen, enabling the geneticist to be confident as to the locus s/he is dealing with. However, this is unusual. Demonstration of a clearly pathogenic mutation in the family, in one of the two alternative genes, would allow confident tracking of the faulty gene.

Knowledge that a disease is genetically homogenous (caused by mutations in only one gene) is therefore usually a prerequisite for the use of linkage for diagnostic purposes. Other important diseases showing locus heterogeneity are tuberous sclerosis, an autosomal dominant disorder which is an important cause of seizures and mental handicap in infancy and childhood, and haemophilia, a coagulation defect inherited as an X-linked recessive. The two forms of haemophilia, haemophilia A and B, though clinically indistinguishable, can fortunately be easily differentiated by coagulation factor assays, which show deficiency respectively of factor VIII or factor IX. The two genes involved, though both X-linked, are separate (*F8C*, Xq28; *F9C*, Xq27) and genetically they must therefore be followed using different polymorphic markers (see Case 4.2 above).

In research rather than in the diagnostic setting linkage can be used to determine the chromosomal locus of specific diseases (Box 4.4).

BOX 4.4 LINKAGE MAPPING OF GENETIC DISEASES; GENETIC MAPS

For diagnostic purposes, markers are chosen which are known to lie close to the gene causing a particular disease, since we can be confident that they will be co-inherited with high probability. In a research setting, though, it is possible to use polymorphic markers for the complementary purpose – that of mapping the position of an *unknown* disease gene. For this, polymorphic markers are chosen at random and their inheritance pattern within disease families is compared with the inheritance of the disease itself. For most markers (which will be on different chromosomes from the disease gene), the marker and disease will appear unassociated, but for a marker close to the disease gene, non-random co-inheritance of marker and disease will be seen. By trial and error (perhaps examining 200–300 markers), significant linkage between marker and disease can be shown statistically.

Once linkage to markers in a particular chromosomal region has been shown, it is then usually fairly simple to examine other markers in the same region to narrow down the mapping of the disease gene. There are now thousands of CA repeat markers of known positions on the human genetic map, with the average genetic distance between useful markers being $\theta<0.01$. This in turn allows modern linkage-based diagnosis to be highly accurate, since risks of recombination are low. Indeed, the accuracy of linkage-based diagnosis tends to be limited much more by the precision of the original diagnosis than by risks of recombination (see below).

CASE 4.4
Prenatal exclusion testing

Family tree

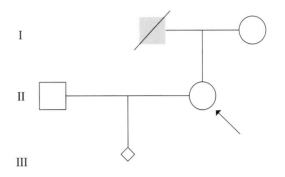

Presenting problem

Hilary, a 30-year-old woman, II-2, has been seen on a number of previous occasions. Her father I-1 died 8 years ago from Huntington's disease (HD), an autosomal dominant condition. Because HD is a late onset disorder, those carrying the mutation may remain asymptomatic until middle age or later. At the age of 30, therefore, Hilary remains at virtually 50% risk of developing HD. In the past, Hilary has enquired about having a presymptomatic test (Chapter 5), to determine whether she herself is carrying the mutation. Because HD is untreatable, she eventually decided against having such a test. However, she is now pregnant.

Although she has not changed her mind about presymptomatic testing, she has a strong desire to ensure that her own future child is not at high risk of HD in the way that she herself is.

What is Huntington's disease?

Huntington's disease is an autosomal dominant neurodegenerative disease in which progressive dementia and an extrapyramidal movement disorder occur. The basal ganglia, particularly the caudate nucleus, show loss of volume on CT or MRI imaging. The disease is one of the group of trinucleotide repeat expansion diseases (see Chapter 8), in which a $(CAG)_n$ sequence within the *HD* gene, encoding polyglutamine in the resulting protein, has become expanded (greater than normal number of triplets) within the affected gene. This type of mutation, because it always affects the same CAG repeat, can be readily tested for in the laboratory. As HD is an autosomal dominant disease, only one of an affected individual's *HD* genes has the mutation. This will be transmitted to offspring with 50% probability.

What has linkage to offer Hilary?

Since the nature of the mutation causing HD is known, it would appear simple to offer prenatal testing to Hilary. However, although detection of the HD mutation would be possible, it would not be desirable in this situation, since if a mutation were found in the fetus, it would also indicate that Hilary herself would develop HD in the future.

Using linkage methods *in preference* to mutation detection, though, it may be possible to exclude the disease in the fetus, without appreciably changing the parent's risk. The results of such an analysis in Hilary's family are shown in Fig. 4.9. A polymorphism known to be very close to the HD gene has been typed.

All the information required for prenatal exclusion testing has been obtained from the two indicated adults (Hilary and her mother). Hilary (II-2) is heterozygous for the HD-linked polymorphism. The *b* allele is clearly the one which she has inherited from her father, but this provides no additional information about her own disease status, since this *b* allele could lie on a normal or an affected paternal chromosome. The fetus has inherited the *a* allele from Hilary. Since this allele comes from Hilary's unaffected mother I-2, the fetus has inherited a *grandmaternal* copy of the *HD* gene, and therefore is at very low risk of developing the disease in future (there will be a small risk of recombination). This constitutes a prenatal exclusion of HD in the fetus. Hilary herself remains at 50% risk. Note that had the fetus inherited her *b* allele, the risk of HD in the fetus would have been 50%, too. Such an outcome would usually result in termination of the pregnancy despite the uncertainty about the fetal disease status; this is the price paid for retaining the uncertainty about the parent's disease status.

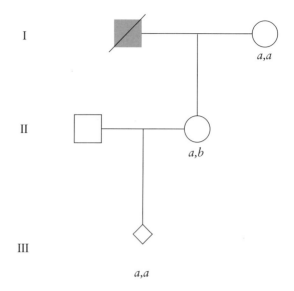

Fig. 4.9 Linkage analysis of Hilary's family using a polymorphic site close to the HD gene.

FURTHER READING

Terwillinger JD, Ott J (1994) *A Handbook of Human Genetic Linkage.* Johns Hopkins University Press.

QUESTIONS (ANSWERS ON PAGE 170)

I If a disease displays allelic heterogeneity
  a linkage analysis cannot be used for diagnosis.
  b mutational analysis cannot help with diagnosis.
  c more than one gene is known to be involved in the disease.
  d autosomal recessive inheritance is rare because homozygosity is unlikely.
  e different mutations may result in different degrees of severity.

2 DNA polymorphisms
  a are present on all chromosomes.
  b can be used to map the genome.
  c can be used to confirm a suspected diagnosis of achondroplasia.
  d can only be typed using restriction endonucleases.
  e can only be typed using DNA from the tissue involved in the disease in question.

3 Variable number tandem repeat polymorphisms (VNTRs)

   a tend to be more informative than RFLPs.

   b are too few in number to be generally useful diagnostically.

   c show high mutation rates.

   d can be used to demonstrate non-paternity in a legal case.

   e can have heterozygosities greater than 90%.

4 Polymorphisms

   a DNA polymorphisms only occur within the introns of genes.

   b Protein polymorphisms are not seen in healthy individuals.

   c If a man is heterozygous for a polymorphism present in the population with an allele frequency of 0.1, the chance of his son having the same polymorphism is 0.05.

   d Some polymorphisms are visible cytogenetically.

   e In a case of Down syndrome, polymorphisms can be used to determine in which parent non-disjunction occurred.

5 Crossing over

   a may result in an error if mutation analysis is being used for prenatal diagnosis.

   b can always be detected if the polymorphism being used to track a disease gene is informative enough.

   c occurs in female but not male meiosis.

   d does not occur on the X chromosome.

   e occurs at the same sites on the chromosome in each meiosis.

6 The following are true of diagnosis by use of linked markers

   a Non-paternity within the family under study may lead to an error in diagnosis.

   b Index case material may be needed before diagnosis in a relative is possible.

   c Use of intragenic polymorphisms gives low risks of error due to recombination.

   d The disease diagnosis must be certain before undertaking a linkage study.

   e Allelic heterogeneity in a disease renders the use of linkage based diagnosis insecure.

7 The following diseases are known to display locus heterogeneity

   a Polycystic kidney disease.

   b Tuberous sclerosis.

   c Cystic fibrosis.

   d Huntington's disease.

   e Duchenne muscular dystrophy.

5

Population Screening and Presymptomatic Testing for Genetic Disease

LEARNING OBJECTIVES

After studying this chapter, the reader should understand:

- the theoretical basis of neonatal screening programmes
- the methods used for predictive testing
- the difficulties in presymptomatic testing for untreatable adult conditions
- particular difficulties in testing children

INTRODUCTION

Medical screening programmes are generally used to identify individuals with a condition for which there is a beneficial medical or lifestyle intervention available. Screening for genetic diseases can be performed at different levels:

- **National** – a successful population-based approach is neonatal screening for phenylketonuria (PKU) (Case 5.1) and congenital hypothyroidism.
- **At-risk populations** – this is a more targeted approach to screening used in particular at-risk groups in the population, such as the programme to identify carriers of Tay–Sachs disease in the Jewish communities in the US and Europe.
- **Families** – determining the disease status of at-risk relatives in families with certain inherited conditions can reduce morbidity and mortality by avoiding environmental triggering factors (Case 5.2) or treating early disease complications (Case 5.3, see also Chapter 9).

- **Individual presymptomatic genetic testing** – determining affected status in an individual before symptoms become apparent. Identification of the molecular basis of untreatable genetic disorders has made presymptomatic testing possible where no medical benefit to early diagnosis exists. Presymptomatic testing does, however, allow the individual to make future lifestyle choices. Predictive genetic testing in this situation has produced a variety of ethical problems (Case 5.4).

In the future DNA-based tests which quantify lifetime risk of common disorders such as ischaemic heart disease, alcoholism, schizophrenia, Alzheimer's disease and diabetes may also become available. Experience with rare genetic disorders should provide a model for an effective and ethical approach to presymptomatic testing.

Some requirements for any screening programme are already apparent:

● the informed participation of individuals should be a primary goal
● information about the rationale and goals of the test must be available to all involved
● an effective system should be in place to do the test and process the results
● the ability to contact individuals with positive results and provide rapid access to medical management and/or counselling is vital.

CASE 5.1
Neonatal screening for phenylketonuria (PKU)

Family tree

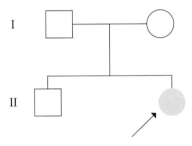

Presenting problem

At the age of 7 days Nicola had a blood sample taken from a heel prick as part of a national neonatal screening program (**Box 5.1**) and following this she was diagnosed as having phenylketonuria (PKU) (Fig. 5.1, **Box 5.2**). Nicola was then referred to the local specialist paediatric metabolic clinic where she was started on a phenylalanine-restricted diet which she has continued. Nicola is now 15 years old and wishes to know what implications PKU has for any children she may have in the future.

Why screen for PKU?

PKU is an autosomal recessive disorder with a UK birth incidence of ~1 in 10 000, and is caused by mutations in the gene encoding the enzyme phenylalanine hydroxylase (PAH) on chromosome 12. PAH converts the amino acid phenylalanine into

tyrosine. Deficiency of this enzyme results in an accumulation of phenylalanine and its metabolites which are toxic to the developing brain. The initial diagnosis was made by detecting an unusually high phenylalanine level (>1200 µmol l^{-1} cf. normal 40–120 µmol l^{-1}) in the dried blood spot from Nicola (**Box 5.2**). If it remains untreated PKU results in severe mental retardation. Treatment involves restriction of dietary phenylalanine by reducing the intake of natural protein and the use of synthetic phenylalanine-free amino acid supplementation. The prognosis for normal intellectual development in PKU is excellent providing treatment is started *early* (within 2 weeks of birth) and the blood phenylalanine levels are well controlled. Parents of a child with PKU are carriers of the condition and therefore have a 1 in 4 recurrence risk for each subsequent pregnancy. Prenatal diagnosis is possible by DNA analysis.

What are the reproductive risks for Nicola?

Nicola is a homozygote for the mutant PAH gene and if the population carrier rate is 1 in 50, then the risk of her future children having PKU can be calculated as follows:

● Nicola's chance of passing on a PKU chromosome is 100% = 1 (Nicola must pass on a copy of the mutated PKU gene as she has no normal PKU gene)
● and her partner's chance of passing on a PKU chromosome = 1/50 × 1/2=1/100 (he has a 1/50 population risk of being a carrier and, if he is a carrier, he has a 1/2 risk of passing on the mutated PKU gene)

Multiplying the risk of both partners therefore gives a combined risk of 1 (Nicola's risk) × 1/100 (partner's risk), i.e. 1/100 for each pregnancy. The risk is obviously higher if she marries a blood relative, as he is more likely to be a carrier, or if she marries a PKU-affected partner, as then all the children must have PKU.

However, it has become apparent that all children of women with PKU are at risk of severe mental and physical developmental damage (especially microcephaly and heart defects) if exposed to high levels of phenylalanine *in utero*. As the fetal

BOX 5.1 NATIONAL NEONATAL SCREENING PROGRAMME

In countries where most births occur under some form of medical supervision, population-based neonatal screening has become routine. The criteria used to decide whether a particular disease is suitable for inclusion in a neonatal screening programme are:

♦ the testing method for that disorder must be sensitive (low false negative rate) and specific (low false positive rate)

♦ effective therapy or intervention must be available

♦ it must be possible to evaluate the outcome and impact of the testing programme in medical social and economic terms

Neonatal screening programmes must be designed for the local population since many genetic conditions show very marked differences in birth incidence between populations. For example, sickle cell disease (E6V mutation in β-globin) occurs at a high rate in many populations of African descent but is rare in caucasians; hepatorenal tyrosinaemia (fumarylacetoacetate hydroxylase deficiency) is very rare in general but more common in French-Canadians; Gaucher's disease type I (glucocerebrosidase deficiency) is common in Ashkenazi Jewish populations. PKU screening is discussed in **Box 5.2** and a non-exhaustive list of other neonatal screening programmes is shown in Table 5.1 below.

Table 5.1 Neonatal screening programmes

Disorder	Birth incidence	Test method	Features	Intervention
Cystic fibrosis	1:2500	Raised immunoreactive trypsin levels or gene mutation analysis	Meconium ileus, recurrent chest infections, failure to thrive	Early physiotherapy, pancreatic enzyme supplements, genetic counselling
Galactosaemia	1:30 000	Reduced galactose-1-phosphate uridyltransferase activity	Mental retardation, cataracts, liver disease	Galactose-free diet
Congenital hypothyroidism*	1:4000	Raised thyroid stimulating hormone	Mental retardation, constipation, failure to thrive	Thyroid hormone replacement
Sickle cell disease	~1:4000 (in afro-caribbeans)	Haemoglobin electrophoresis	Stroke, bone pain, pneumococcal infections	Penicillin prophylaxis, pain relief
Maple syrup urine disease	1:180 000	Raised branch-chain amino acids levels	Vomiting, acidosis, seizures, mental handicap	Restrict intake of branch-chain amino acids in diet
Biotinidase deficiency	<1:100 000	Biotinidase activity	Vomiting, seizures, ataxia, skin rash	High-dose biotin

*Currently offered in Scotland with PKU screening.

phenylalanine level is dependent on maternal phenylalanine metabolism, this risk occurs independent of whether the fetus has inherited PKU or not. For this reason Nicola will therefore be advised to plan her pregnancies carefully and maintain a very strict control of her blood phenylalanine levels both in the periconceptual period and throughout pregnancy.

BOX 5.2 SCREENING FOR PKU ON DRIED BLOOD SPOTS

Heel-prick blood samples are collected by the hospital or community midwife on to absorbent card (Guthrie card) at ~6 days post delivery (collection of blood into glass capillary tubes is used as an alternative in some regions). The test is performed at 6 days because normal feeding is likely to have been established and a normal amount of protein (and, therefore, phenylalanine) will have been consumed. The Guthrie cards are sent to a central testing facility where the blood-filled discs are placed on an agar plate which has been seeded with bacteria that require the amino acid phenylalanine for growth. Since the phenylalanine level in blood is normally low, only bacteria surrounding a sample with an abnormally high level will be able to grow (Fig. 5.1). This technique is semiquantitative and relatively inexpensive. There is now over 30 years' experience in the UK of neonatal screening for PKU by this means and it has proven to be both a clinically beneficial and cost-effective exercise.

An abnormal test result is immediately reported to the local specialist paediatrician and dietician and they will usually see the child within 24 h to confirm the diagnosis and start the appropriate treatment.

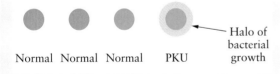

Normal   Normal   Normal   PKU

Halo of bacterial growth

Fig. 5.1 Neonatal testing for PKU.

CASE 5.2
Testing for genetic susceptibility to environmental agents

Family tree

Presenting problem

Phyllis (II-1) and her younger sister Margo (II-4) were referred to the genetic clinic by a consultant psychiatrist. Phyllis had recently been admitted as an emergency with an acute psychotic episode from which she has completely recovered. Their brother (II-3) and mother (I-2) had both died of unexplained illnesses after emergency abdominal surgery. Phyllis has had occasional bouts of acute abdominal pain and her father has demanded that someone 'gets to the bottom of' the family problems. On investigation a sample of Phyllis' urine showed increased levels of porphobilinogen, and subsequent red cell porphobilinogen deaminase (PBGD) enzyme assay showed a ~50% reduction from normal level. A diagnosis of acute intermittent porphyria (AIP) was made.

What is the mechanism of the disease in AIP?

AIP is a rare autosomal dominant disorder affecting ~1 in 50 000 and caused by mutations in the PBGD gene on chromosome 11q24. PBGD is an enzyme involved in the complex synthesis of haem molecules. Symptoms of AIP are very rare before puberty but in adults include abdominal discomfort, vomiting, paralysis, seizures, psychotic episodes and hypertension. These decompensation symptoms are triggered by environmental factors, the most common being drugs (e.g. barbiturates, sulphonamides), alcohol, infections and hormonal changes. All of these environmental triggers are

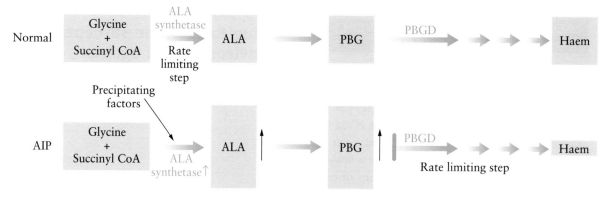

Fig. 5.2 The biochemical basis of AIP. RLS=rate-limiting step (least efficient step in the metabolic process).

thought to increase the activity of aminolevulinic acid (ALA) synthase activity in the liver. In the normal situation 50% PBGD activity is sufficient to prevent the build-up of toxic precursors in the haem synthesis pathway. However if there is an increase in ALA synthetase activity, which is normally the rate-limiting step in the pathway, a pathological accumulation of intermediates occurs for which the PBGD activity cannot compensate (Fig. 5.2).

What treatment is available?

As with all genetic conditions with environmentally triggered crises (**Box 5.3**) the avoidance of precipitating factors is the mainstay of management in AIP. All affected individuals should wear bracelets or carry a card warning of their condition. It is likely that individuals I-2 and II-3 died as a result of unnecessary exploratory operations for abdominal pain. During the acute attack, analgesia, withdrawal of precipitating agent and supportive therapy are currently the best approach.

What is the implication of Phyllis's diagnosis for Margo?

As the diagnosis of AIP has been made in Phyllis, Margo, who is still too young to be symptomatic, can be screened by measuring her PBGD activity to see whether or not she is also affected. If affected, prophylactic advice will help her avoid triggering symptoms.

CASE 5.3
Adult polycystic kidney disease (APKD)

Family tree

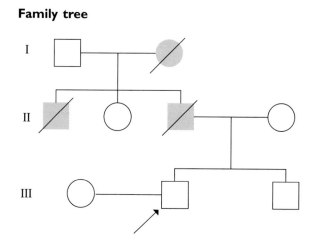

Presenting problem

Andrew (III-2) is 25 years old and has been referred to the genetic clinic because he has recently become engaged and wishes to know if he has inherited adult polycystic kidney disease (APKD) present in his family. This condition had been diagnosed in the family after his father died of a cerebral haemorrhage at the age of 43 years. A post-mortem examination revealed that he had a ruptured berry aneurysm and bilateral multiple renal cysts. Andrew's paternal uncle (II-1) and grandmother (I-2) had both died in their 50s with chronic renal failure, their death certificates revealing a diagnosis of 'polycystic kidneys'. A recent renal ultrasound on Andrew was normal.

BOX 5.3 GENETIC DISORDERS WITH ENVIRONMENTAL TRIGGER

It has been known for many years that some individuals experience unusual and often dangerous responses to certain drugs. The discovery that there is a genetic basis to many of the non-immunological reactions to pharmacological agents has provided one of the few successes in prevention of mortality and morbidity in genetic disorders. In most of these conditions simple avoidance of exposure to specific environmental triggering events is sufficient to prevent disease.

◆ **Malignant hyperpyrexia (MH)** – in some families is caused by mutations in the ryanodine receptor gene on chromosome 19q13, affects ~1 in 15 000. MH causes potentially fatal reactions to halogenated volatile anaesthetic agents resulting in muscle stiffness, myoglobinuria and extreme pyrexia which are caused by the excessive release of ionized calcium from the sarcoplasmic reticulum of skeletal muscle. Although the disorder is now treatable with a drug called Dantrolene, there is still a significant mortality rate. MH is an autosomal dominant condition and all first-degree relatives of an affected individual should be investigated in specialist centres by exposing a biopsied muscle fragment to caffeine and halothane. Susceptible individuals have muscles with an abnormally high contractile response to these agents. These individuals should carry a card or bracelet warning of this susceptibility and all involved health professionals must then be advised of the specific triggering agents to be avoided

◆ **Butyrylcholinesterase deficiency** – caused by mutations in the butyrylcholinesterase gene on chromosome 3q26, affects ~1 in 3000 people. This condition causes susceptibility to the actions of succinylcholine (a muscle relaxant with rapid onset of action used at the beginning of anaesthesia to enable endotracheal intubation) producing prolonged paralysis. It is an autosomal recessive condition and testing 'at-risk' individuals is done by measuring the percentage inhibition of plasma cholinesterase activity by dibucaine (an amide-type local anaesthetic)

◆ **G-6-PD deficiency** – caused by mutations in the glucose-6-phosphate dehydrogenase gene on chromosome Xq28, is one of the commonest genetic disorders worldwide. Although it is rare in caucasian populations, it is common in people of African and Mediterranean descent. It produces a drug-induced haemolytic anaemia with many agents, including nalidixic acid and primaquin and is also called favism because of a haemolytic response to eating fava beans.

◆ **Acute intermittent porphyria** – see Case 5.2.

What causes APKD?

APKD is a relatively common autosomal dominant disease with an incidence of ~1 in 1000 in the population. The disease shows genetic locus heterogeneity, with mutations in the polycystin gene on chromosome 16p13 causing the condition in ~95% of families and the remaining ~5% of families having a mutation in an unknown gene on chromosome 4q21.

Why screen relatives of affected individuals for APKD?

APKD is characterized by the development of destructive renal cysts (~10% of patients in renal dialysis programmes in the UK have APKD) and intracranial aneurysms. There is considerable variability in disease penetrance with ~50% of individuals with APKD being asymptomatic. However, ~50% of asymptomatic gene carriers have treatable complications such as hypertension and early renal failure, and it is thought that the early diagnosis of the condition reduces morbidity and mortality associated with these complications.

Has Andrew inherited the APKD gene?

Even with the problem of locus heterogeneity mentioned above, it is possible to establish linkage to chromosomes 16p or 4q in large families, which can then be used to determine an individual's risk (see Chapter 4). However, in Andrew's family there is no DNA available from any of the affected individuals, and therefore DNA testing is not available. In this situation phenotypic investigation is used to help establish genetic status (**Box 5.4**). Renal ultrasound scanning to detect renal cysts is the most common method used for phenotypic testing in APKD (Fig. 5.3). However, the reassurance given by a normal renal scan is dependent on the age at which the screening is performed. It is known that ~86% of APKD gene carriers will develop renal cysts by the age of 25, and therefore a normal renal scan before this age gives less reassurance than one obtained after this age. A Bayesian calculation (Table 5.2) can be used to combine the reassurance given by Andrew's normal renal ultrasound scan at age 25, with his prior genetic risk (1 in 2) to give an overall likelihood of ~1 in 8 that he carries the mutated APKD gene despite a normal scan (See Chapter 7, Case 7.3 for explanation of Bayesian risk analysis).

Phenotypic testing will be unable to give Andrew complete reassurance that he does not carry the gene, as non-penetrance in this condition means that 1 in 7 gene carriers of APKD show no signs of the disease. Thus for complete reassurance a genetic test is required which excludes mutations from both APKD genes, and such a test is not yet available.

Table 5.2 Bayesian calculation of risk

Bayesian calculation	Carrier	Non-carrier
Prior risk	0.5	0.5
Conditional risk (negative renal ultrasound)	0.14	1
Joint risk (prior × conditional)	0.07	0.5
Posterior	0.07/(0.5+0.07) = 0.12=~1 in 8	0.5/(0.5+0.07) =0.88=~7 in 8

(a)

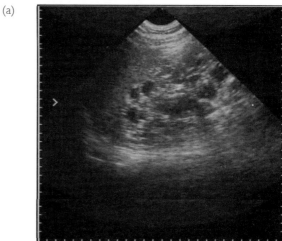

(b)

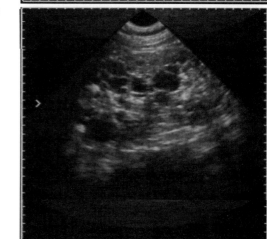

Fig. 5.3 Ultrasound showing multiple renal cysts in a patient with adult polycystic kidney disease. (a) Left kidney; (b) right kidney. (Figure supplied by Dr A Stevenson.)

BOX 5.4 PHENOTYPIC TESTING FOR GENETIC DISEASE

Phenotypic testing involves the search for specific clinical signs present before the onset of symptoms which enable the assignment of affected status to an individual. This type of testing is particularly useful in adult onset genetic disorders where useful clinical intervention is possible but the molecular basis of the disease is not understood or is not easily determined. One major disadvantage of phenotypic testing is that although it allows the unequivocal determination of affected status, it is often more difficult to confirm that an individual has not inherited the mutant gene. This is due to the phenomenon of non-penetrance seen in many autosomal dominant disorders, where the gene can be 'carried' by a phenotypically normal individual (Chapter 1). APKD (Case 5.3), familial hypercholesterolaemia and hypertrophic obstructive cardiomyopathy (HOCM) are examples of genetic diseases where phenotypic presymptomatic testing is widely used.

CASE 5.4
Cascade screening for cystic fibrosis

Family tree

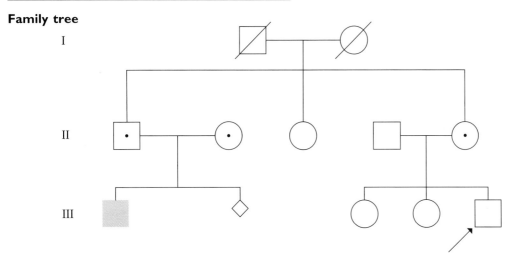

Presenting problem

This family has previously been discussed in Chapter 4, Case 4.1. Josh (III-5) is 18 years old and has been contacted by the local genetics department as part of a cascade screening programme for cystic fibrosis (CF). His cousin, Robert (III-1), was diagnosed as having CF at the age of 2½ years and is heterozygous for the ΔF508 mutation in the CFTR gene (see Chapter 4, Fig 4.1). This mutation can be detected using a PCR assay (Chapter 3, Box 3.4) or amplification refractory mutation analysis (ARMS, **Box 5.5**). ARMS is most conveniently performed on DNA extracted from the buccal cells in a mouth wash specimen. Josh's maternal uncle (II-1) and mother (II-5) have sent a mouthwash to the laboratory and have been found to carry this mutation. Josh has been offered the same test.

What is cascade screening?

Cascade screening differs from population-based screening in that the offer of genetic testing is targeted to the relatives of affected individuals. This type of screening is most suitable for X-linked recessive disorders such as Fragile X and common autosomal recessive disorders such as cystic fibrosis. The advantage of this system is the high pick-up rate for mutation detection in relatives, therefore fewer tests are performed to pick up a carrier than in a population-based approach. The disadvantages in autosomal recessive disorders are:

- This approach is unlikely to pick up most couples who are at 1 in 4 risk of having an affected child, since there is no known family history in most new cases of autosomal recessive disorders.
- Knowledge of carrier status is not usually useful unless:
- reproduction is an issue and there is an accurate test available to determine the genetic status of the partner.
- there is specific lifestyle measures that will avoid a deleterious effect of carrier status, e.g. smoking and α1-antitrypsin deficiency.

What is the benefit of this screening test to Josh?

Josh is young, healthy and unattached. He currently has no plans to have children and, as there is no (non-reproductive) health advantage to knowing carrier status, after discussing the situation with a genetic counsellor he decided not to have the test at the present time. He will contact the department for a couple screen if and when he decides to have children.

BOX 5.5 ARMS TESTING

This system relies on the fact that the 3' end of PCR primers must match the target DNA exactly to allow amplification. Thus primers can be manufactured that will assay for the presence of the normal allele and the mutant allele. Using such a system allows the laboratory to determine the genetic status of an individual for any single-base mutation or small deletion.

Figure 5.4a shows two possible alleles at a given locus which differ by a single nucleotide, a C in allele 1 and a T in the same position in allele 2. Primer A has a C at its 3' end corresponding to the variable site, whereas primer B has a T and is longer. Primer C is a common primer that will amplify with either A or B. If allele 1 is present then primers A and C will amplify a fragment of 205 base-pairs (bp), if allele 2 is present then primers B and C will amplify a fragment of 220 bp. The genetic status can be determined by electrophoresing the PCR products and staining the DNA bands (Fig. 5.4b)

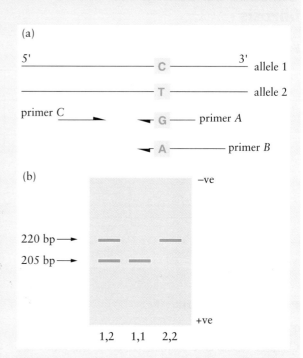

Fig. 5.4 (a) Two possible alleles which differ by a single nucleotide. (b) Separation of PCR products by electrophoresis. The first lane shows heterozygosity while lanes 2 and 3 indicate homozygosity for alleles 1 and 2, respectively.

What is a couple screen ?

Couple screening is an approach to identify couples at 1 in 4 risk of having a child with a severe autosomal recessive disorder with particular advantages in CF. In Josh's case, he has a 50% chance of being a carrier of ΔF508 mutation and in most circumstances his future partner will have a population risk of carrying any CF mutation, i.e. ~1 in 20. In northern European populations ~85% of all CF gene mutations can be detected using an ARMS assay for four different mutations: ΔF508, G551D, G542X and 621+1G→T. The couple screen reports a specific risk only if both partners are found to be carrier since in this situation accurate prenatal or postnatal diagnosis would be possible.

Thus if Josh was found to be a carrier and his partner was not, they would be reported as a low-risk of having a pregnancy affected with CF. The actual risk could be calculated:

Joshs' risk of being a carrier = 1 multiplied by partner's risk of being a carrier

= prior risk (population carrier frequency) × partner's negative ARMS screen risk (ARMS only detects 85% of mutations so there is a 15% risk that an undetected mutation is still present)

= 1/20 × 3/20 = 3/400

multiplied by
risk of affected child if both were carriers
(1 in 4) = **1 in 533.**

Although this is higher than the population risk
it is a low risk and no useful prenatal testing would
be available. If an ARMS test was available that
could detect 95% of CF mutations then a negative
test on Josh's partner would reduce the risk to 1
in 1600 (population risk).

Although couple screening can be very useful, it
is important that the participants realize that the
risk of having an affected child is reduced but not
eliminated. Adequate counselling services must
also be available for couples who are found to be
at 1 in 4 risk.

CASE 5.5
Presymptomatic testing for Huntington's disease

Family tree

Presenting problem

Senga (III-2) is 22 years old and wishes to know
whether she has inherited the gene for Huntington's
disease which affects her father Jim (II-5).

What is Huntington's Disease ?

Huntington's Disease (HD) is an autosomal dominant condition caused by expansion of a trinucleotide repeat in the HD gene on chromosome
4p16.3 (Chapter 8, Box 8.1). HD affects ~1 in
10 000 people with an average age of onset of
35 years. Clinically it is characterized by progressive involuntary movements (chorea), weight loss,
psychiatric symptoms and progressive dementia.
On neuropathological examination, atrophy of the
caudate nucleus is typical and can also be detected
in vivo using CT or MRI scan of brain (Fig. 5.5).
There is currently no effective therapy for HD and
the average time between diagnosis and death is
15 years.

Why test asymptomatic individuals?

There are many untreatable, late-onset genetic
diseases. Requests for genetic advice come from
knowledgeable family members who are at risk
of developing the condition themselves. There is
often a demand from within these families for

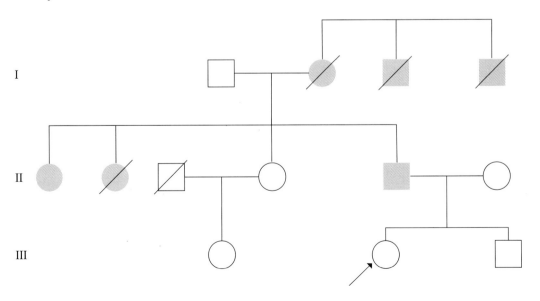

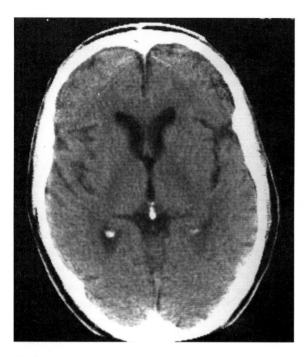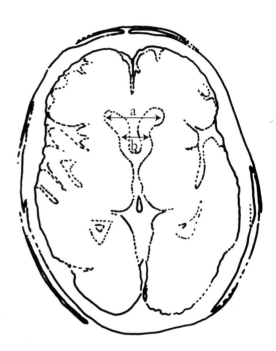

Fig. 5.5 CT scan of patient with HD showing caudate atrophy resulting in variation in shape of lateral ventricles. This can be quantified as a decrease in the ratio a/b. (Figure supplied by Dr Robin Sellar.)

presymptomatic testing (PST), in order to detect inheritance of the mutant gene before the onset of disease. There are several different reasons given for requesting PST in untreatable genetic disease:

● to make decisions about having children
● to clarify the risk to existing offspring
● to plan future health needs
● inability to cope with the uncertainty of not knowing

Advances in molecular genetics have made the accurate prediction of genetic status possible in certain diseases where there is no means of treatment or prevention. It is now widely accepted that at-risk individuals have a right to know their genetic status even if there is no medical advantage in this knowledge. However, this situation does present particular ethical problems for family members and clinicians.

How is the test structured?

The majority of people who enter a PST programme wish to have their belief confirmed that they have not inherited the disorder. Unfortunately, ~50% will find out that they are going to develop an untreatable disorder, and as a corollary that their children are now at 50% risk of inheriting the same condition. Considerable care has been taken in the development of testing procedures so as to minimize the problems inherent in PST.

● **Age** – individuals entering PST should be adults. Testing of children is not usually recommended as such testing for an adult-onset untreatable condition conveys no medical advantage to the child. Parents have a duty to, but no rights over, their children, each child has the prerogative to make their own decision about PST at a later date when they can comprehend its implications.
● **Autonomy** – in PST for untreatable disorders, where no clinical intervention is possible, there is no medical reason for having the test. The wishes of the individual to be tested are paramount, and undue pressure from any outside agency, relative or partner should be discouraged.
● **Thinking time** – counselling sessions are recommended at spaced intervals before the test to allow the at-risk individual to consider the full implications of gaining knowledge that cannot later be 'unlearned'.

● **Coping procedures** – an adequate social support network should be organized and a plan formulated for the period after a positive result is known. A negative result can also be problematic, engendering a large degree of guilt especially where other members of the family have tested positive.

If the at-risk individual makes an informed decision to have the test, it should be carried out with the minimum of delay and there should be a detailed plan for disclosing the results and post-test follow-up.

What specific issues are important in PST counselling?

Three counselling sessions were arranged for Senga, covering the following main issues:
● the genetic risk of inheriting the gene for HD (in Senga's case 1 in 2)
● information on the clinical features of HD.
● implications of a positive test result are:

● the individual tested will develop HD (although prediction of the age of onset of clinical symptoms is not currently possible)
● the risk to offspring of the individual increases to 1 in 2
● insurance companies may penalize known gene carriers
● regulations may forbid the issue of immigration visa to some countries

What was the outcome of PST for Senga?

Senga decided to undergo PST and had the DNA test. Analysis of the $(CAG)_n$ repeat (**Box 5.6** and Chapter 8, Box 8.1) showed that Senga has inherited the gene for HD from her father and will therefore develop HD. When Senga received the result, 2 weeks after the blood test was taken, she was distraught. However, when seen at several follow-up appointments, Senga said that she did not regret having the test despite the difficulties in coming to terms with the results. She finds that the

---

BOX 5.6 $(CAG)_n$ REPEAT EXPANSION MUTATIONS

Several different autosomal dominant neurological disorders have been found to be due to expansion mutations in a $(CAG)_n$ repeat:

◆ **Kennedy disease** – spinobulbar muscular atrophy, an X-linked condition with onset of muscle weakness and wasting, usually in middle age, caused by expansion of $(CAG)_n$ repeats within the androgen receptor gene.
◆ **Spinocerebellar ataxia type I (SCA I)** – late-onset cerebellar ataxia with dementia caused by an expanded repeat in the ataxin gene on chromosome 6p.
◆ **Spinocerebellar ataxia type III (SCA III)** – also known as Machado–Joseph disease, late-onset cerebellar ataxia with dementia caused by repeat expansion on chromosome 14q.
◆ **Dentatorubropallidoluysian atrophy** – choreoathetosis, myoclonic epilepsy and dementia caused by a repeat expansion in the B37 gene

on chromosome 12p.
◆ **Huntington's disease** – see Case 5.4.
◆ **Myotonic dystrophy** – see Chapter 8, Case 8.2.

In all of these disorders, where a large number of cases are examined the number of $(CAG)_n$ repeats is indirectly proportional to the age of onset of clinical features. However, this association is only significant in very large alleles and is not sufficient to give accurate advice about likely age-of-onset to individual patients. Abnormally large $(CAG)_n$ repeats appear to be relatively unstable in meiosis, and significant intergenerational increases in allele size may occur, particularly in male meiosis in HD. This phenomenon is the basis of anticipation, i.e. the clinical observation that as the condition is passed down through the generations, it becomes more severe and occurs at an increasingly younger age (see Chapter 8, Case 8.2).

test result occupies her mind for a large portion of each day, but she has gradually been able to get back to her usual working and social routines.

What about other members of her family?

After Senga had her result, Gloria (III-1) contacted the clinical genetics department to request PST. Gloria's mother is clinically unaffected at the age of 52, and does not wish to have a predictive test. This situation presents a particular ethical problem. If Gloria, who is 30 years old and is at a 1 in 4 genetic risk, has the test which shows her to be a gene carrier, she has effectively established that her mother is also a carrier, as Gloria must have inherited her affected grandmother's gene through her own mother. Current practice however supports Gloria's right to know her own genetic status, even if her mother does not wish to know hers. After counselling, Gloria had PST which showed that she had not inherited her grandmother's mutated gene. Gloria's mother, however, remains at a 1 in 2 risk of having her own mother's (Gloria's grandmother's) mutated gene.

FURTHER READING

Andrews LB, Fullarton JE, Holtzman NA, Motulsky AG (eds) (1994) *Assessing Genetic Risk*. National Academy Press, Washington DC.

Harper PS (1993) *Practical Genetic Counselling*, 4th edn. Butterworth Heinemann, Oxford.

QUESTIONS (ANSWERS ON PAGE 171)

1 Neonatal screening for biochemical genetic disorders
a is best done in the first 24 h of life.
b became widely available in the UK in the 1980s.
c is most often performed on urine samples.
d takes ~1 month for result to be available.
e is organized by individual hospitals.

2 Huntington's disease is
a associated with caudate atrophy.
b often diagnosed in childhood.
c often associated with psychiatric symptoms.
d has a mean age of onset of 55 years.
e predictable by DNA testing.

3 Adult polycystic kidney disease (APKD)
a is symptomatic in ~50% of cases.
b has an incidence of 1 in 100 000 births.
c is caused by mutations in at least two different loci.
d is associated with cerebral aneurysm formation.
e is a relatively common cause of end-stage renal failure.

4 Acute intermittent porphyria (AIP)
a is an autosomal recessive disorder.
b may be triggered by infections.
c is caused by deficiency of ALA synthetase.
d is a common cause of acute psychosis.
e can be diagnosed on urine testing.

5 Drug-induced decompensation is a feature of the following disorders:
a Malignant hyperpyrexia
b Glucose-6-phosphate dehydrogenase deficiency
c Tay–Sachs disease
d C1 esterase inhibitor deficiency
e butyrylcholinesterase deficiency.

6 Phenylketonuria
a causes accumulation of tyrosine in the plasma.
b biochemically improves with age.
c usually presents at ~2 months of age.
d is commonly associated with microcephaly and heart defects.
e in untreated cases causes fair hair and blue eyes.

7 Presymptomatic testing in genetic diseases by DNA analysis
a should only be performed where adequate treatment is available.
b can only be done in individuals at 50% risk.
c must never be done in children.
d requires consent.
e is possible in familial cancer syndromes.

8 Phenotypic testing in genetic diseases

  a can prevent morbidity.

  b for APKD is best done by abdominal examination.

  c uses DNA analysis.

  d is possible in familial cancer syndromes.

  e is a useful way to exclude carrier status.

6

Prenatal Diagnosis

LEARNING OBJECTIVES

After studying this chapter, the reader should understand:

- the use and limitations of prenatal diagnosis
- the techniques used in prenatal diagnosis
- the principles of screening during pregnancy

INTRODUCTION

Prenatal diagnosis is available for a wide variety of disorders, single gene and chromosomal, as well as for structural abnormalities, either multifactorial or without any genetic aetiology. There are two types of diagnostic procedure: non-invasive, e.g. ultrasound scanning (**Box 6.1**); and invasive, e.g. chorionic villus sampling (CVS, **Box 6.2**), amniocentesis (**Box 6.3**) and fetal blood sampling (**Box 6.4**). The choice of test is to some extent dictated by the condition being investigated, but also involves women and frequently their partners coming to an informed decision about the test they would prefer.

Prenatal diagnosis should be offered with no pre-conditions. In particular, there should be no pressure on the woman to terminate the pregnancy in the event of an abnormal finding, but making a diagnosis of an abnormality in a fetus offers the parents the chance to consider termination of the pregnancy. As well as allowing medical staff time to optimize conditions for delivery of the baby and treatment of the abnormality where no termination takes place, it can also give families prior

warning of possible problems to come so that they can prepare psychologically for the baby's arrival.

There is no prenatal diagnostic test for the majority of single-gene disorders, most of which are very rare. However, for those where the underlying molecular defect is known and the mutation characterized, the pregnancy can be investigated by CVS or amniocentesis (see Chapter 3 and Cases 6.1 and 6.5 in this chapter). In cases where the underlying molecular defect is unknown, but the family has a suitable structure for linkage analysis (see Chapter 4), a high or low risk haplotype or marker pattern can be identified and tested for on DNA obtained at CVS or amniocentesis.

It is important therefore whenever a clinical geneticist sees a patient with a single-gene disorder for which either mutation or linkage analysis is available, s/he should consider the likelihood that a prenatal diagnostic test may in future be requested by a family member. For this reason DNA should be stored and the DNA analysis should be done in advance of a pregnancy so that a prenatal test can be performed swiftly and efficiently.

BOX 6.1 ULTRASOUND SCANNING

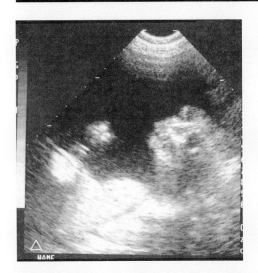

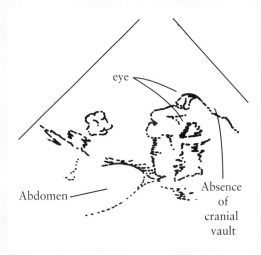

eye

Abdomen

Absence
of
cranial
vault

Fig. 6.1 Prenatal ultrasound of anencephaly. Note the lack of cranium development and associated bulging eyes. (Figure supplied by Dr Lena Macara.)

Ultrasound imaging is based on the pulse-echo principle in which a short burst of sound waves is emitted by a transducer which then picks up the echoes reflected from the structures in the line of the pulse. At 20–24 weeks' gestation a frequency of 5 MHz is used, whilst later in the pregnancy 3.5 MHz is preferred. These echoes are converted to images and displayed on a monitor. Ultrasound is generally regarded as safe and is a very widely used examination technique. Although in the past the vast

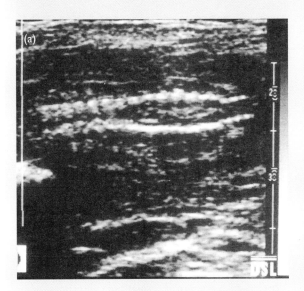

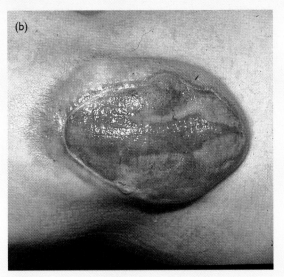

Fig. 6.2 (a) Prenatal ultrasound of a neural tube defect. The arrows show a bony defect where the vertebrae have failed to develop properly. (b) A neural tube defect showing the exposed neural tissue. (c) Neural tube defects are often associated with hydrocephalus which can be seen prenatally by the presence of a 'lemon-shaped' skull and 'banana-shaped' posterior fossa. (Figure 6.2a supplied by Dr Lena Macara; Figure 6.2c supplied by Dr Sarah Chambers.)

BOX 6.1 ULTRASOUND SCANNING (Cont.)

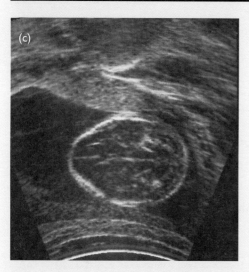

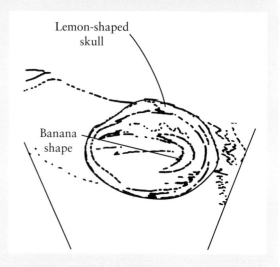

Lemon-shaped skull

Banana shape

majority of women had an ultrasound scan at the clinic booking visit, at 10–12 weeks' gestation, to determine the number of fetuses and the expected date of delivery, there is now evidence suggesting a routine anomaly scan at 18–20 weeks would be more informative.

Ultrasound is particularly useful for identifying many major structural abnormalities classically anencephaly (Fig. 6.1) and spina bifida (Fig. 6.2). However, it has the disadvantage that it can also display features in late gestation scans whose significance is uncertain, such as renal dilatation. This can lead to diagnostic difficulties and increased maternal anxiety.

Recently there has been research in certain centres in combining 'soft markers' seen in ultrasound scanning such as chorioid plexus cysts, nuchal translucency and sandal gap (increased distance between 1st and 2nd toes, Fig. 6.3), with serum screening results for Down syndrome to refine the individual risk of having an affected pregnancy. This is particularly relevant in first trimester screening (**Box 6.7**).

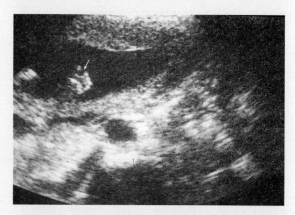

Fig. 6.3 An increased distance between the first and second toe (see arrow) is associated with Downs syndrome. (Figure supplied by Dr Lena Macara.)

BOX 6.2 CHORIONIC VILLUS SAMPLING

◆ Routinely performed at 10–12 weeks' gestation. Very early CVS has been implicated in limb reduction defects. Can be undertaken at 16 weeks in preference to amniocentesis.

◆ Involves sampling of chorion tissue, placental in origin, by insertion of needle under ultrasound guidance. Approach can be trans-abdominal or, less frequently, trans-cervical.

◆ Miscarriage risk approximately 2%, on a background risk at this gestation of 2–4%.

◆ Comprised of syncytiotrophoblasts, outer non-dividing cells, and cytotrophoblasts, rapidly divid-

ing cells (Fig. 6.4). Quantity of sample allows DNA extraction and presence of dividing cells allows fetal karyotyping without prior culturing.

◆ Approximately 1% of karotyping gives rise to mosaic results (Chapter 2, Box 2.4), 70% of which, due to placental origin of the tissue, have no clinical significance. A confirmatory karyotype is always obtained from cultured cells.

◆ Allows measurement of enzyme levels in direct or cultured cells for metabolic disorders.

◆ Care must be taken to avoid maternal tissue contamination.

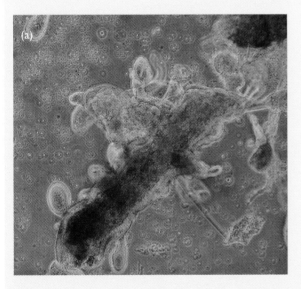

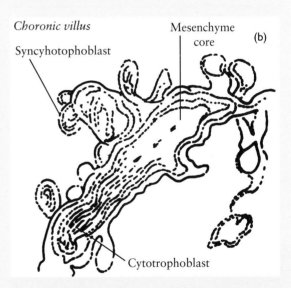

Choronic villus Mesenchyme core (b)

Syncyhotophoblast

Cytotrophoblast

Fig. 6.4 (a) Photograph of chorionic villus. (b) Outline of villus showing outer layer of cells (syncytiotrophoblasts) and inner layer of highly dividing cytotrophoblasts, surrounding a mesenchymal core. (Figure 6.4a supplied by Dr David Gilmore.)

BOX 6.3 AMNIOCENTESIS

◆ Routinely performed at 15–16 weeks' gestation, although there is an increasing trend to perform it at 14 weeks. Earlier procedures, in the first trimester, are technically more difficult because of the small volume of amniotic fluid present, although a closed system is being developed to filter the cells from the amniotic fluid which is then replaced.

◆ Involves removal of 10–20 ml of amniotic fluid by aspiration under ultrasound guidance.

◆ Miscarriage risk approximately 1%.

◆ Comprises fetal urine and cells from different fetal cell lineages, only 20% of which are viable. Few of the cells are actively dividing and therefore culture is required prior to fetal karyotyping or DNA extraction.

◆ Culture delays results by 2–3 weeks but as the majority of cells are of fetal origin, placental mosaicism is less problematic. Recent advances mean that interphase FISH (Chapter 2, Box 2.17, Fig. 2.11) can be used to diagnose Down syndrome within a week.

BOX 6.4 FETAL BLOOD SAMPLING

Fetal blood sampling is performed as an out-patient procedure under local anaesthetic. A needle is inserted under ultrasound guidance into the umbilical vein close to the placental insertion. A blood sample is aspirated and its fetal origin confirmed rapidly by determination of mean cell volume. Fetal red cells are larger than their adult counterparts.

Fetal blood sampling may be useful for investigation of ambiguous karyotype results obtained at amniocentesis, as well as for assessment of the degree of feto-maternal alloimmunization in Rhesus disease. In addition fetal infection in particular with toxoplasmosis can be detected by looking at levels of specific IgM in fetal blood.

CASE 6.1
Ultrasound diagnosis: Jeune syndrome

Family tree

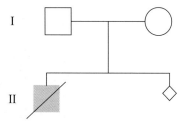

Presenting problem

Helen and her partner Stuart (I-2 and I-1) have been referred for genetic counselling after their first child died at 5 days of age with 'lethal dwarfism'. No post-mortem was carried out. The couple are keen to try for another baby.

What is the recurrence risk for this 'lethal dwarfism'?

'Lethal dwarfism' can arise from a fault in a number of genes. Without a post-mortem diagnosis, it is difficult to determine the gene at fault and to give Helen and Stuart an accurate recurrence risk. Doctors are often reluctant to cause more distress to parents after the death of a baby by asking for a post-mortem. However, without one, a couple will be disadvantaged by the lack of a firm diagnosis, although sometimes photographs and X-rays taken prior to death can give some clues.

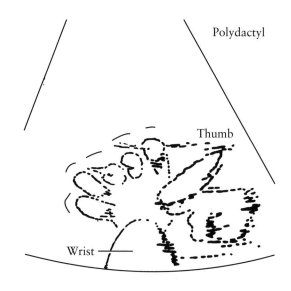

Fig. 6.5 Prenatal ultrasound right hand, palm facing, showing the presence of six fingers (polydactyl) with the thumb on the right of the picture. (Figure supplied by Dr Lena Macara.)

What diagnostic tests are available for a future pregnancy?

Ultrasound scanning can be helpful in the detection of severe prenatal skeletal abnormalities. When Helen again became pregnant, she was offered a dating scan (**Box 6.1**) and further scans every 2 weeks from 14 weeks of pregnancy to assess fetal growth. At 16 weeks the radiologist became concerned by the abnormally bright echo pattern seen in the fetal kidneys. Polydactyly (extra digits) (Fig. 6.5) of the right hand and foot were noted, in conjunction with a small chest size. A tentative diagnosis of Jeune syndrome was made, and the findings discussed with the couple who opted to terminate the pregnancy based on this information.

What is Jeune syndrome?

Jeune syndrome is an autosomal recessive condition that affects skeletal growth, in particular the chest wall, and usually leads to death from respiratory failure in infancy. As in this case, it can be associated with polydactyly. The kidneys are also affected, and children who survive the neonatal period almost invariably develop renal failure in childhood. The diagnosis can be confirmed at post-mortem on the basis of characteristic bone histology (Fig. 6.6) and X-ray appearance (Fig. 6.7).

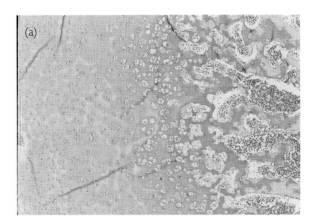

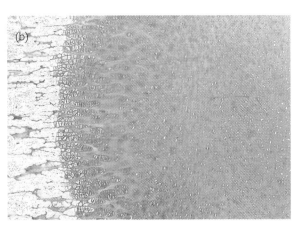

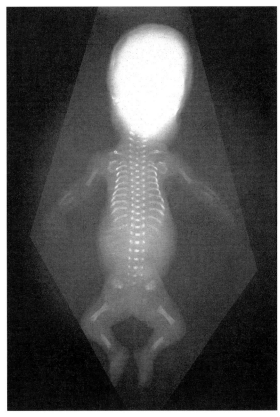

Fig. 6.7 X-ray of fetus with Jeune syndrome. Note short limbs. (Figure supplied by Dr Nick Smith.)

Fig. 6.6 (a) Characteristic bone histology found in Jeune syndrome. Note irregular cartilage–bone junction.
(b) Normal bone histology with smooth cartilage–bone junction. (Figures supplied by Dr Alan Howatson.)

CASE 6.2
X-linked mental retardation

Family tree

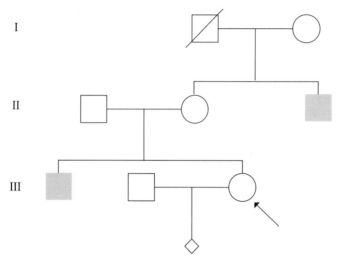

Presenting problem

Jane (III-3) is 26 years old and 10 weeks' pregnant. She informs the midwife that she has a brother, Alan, with 'mental handicap', and would like pre-natal diagnosis to make sure that she does not have a child with a similar problem. Both Alan and their maternal uncle, who appears to be similarly affected, have been seen and investigated by the local genetics department 3 years previously and a diagnosis of X-linked mental retardation was made.

What should the midwife do?

As Jane is already 10 weeks' pregnant, it is impor-tant that all available facts on the condition in the family are reviewed promptly. Is there good evi-dence from the history and clinical examination that Alan and his uncle have the same condition, and if so, does it resemble any of the known X-linked mental retardation phenotypes? Has Alan had a recent chromosome analysis and has he been tested for Fragile X syndrome? Urgent contact should be made with the genetics department to resolve these issues and confirm that there are no new tests available which should be offered.

What did these investigations elicit?

Alan has a normal karyotype and tested negative for Fragile X syndrome (Chapter 8). Neither he nor his uncle have any specific dysmorphic features, but both have a similar pattern of severe learning difficulties and hyperactivity. Jane tells the midwife that her mother's life has been made a misery by caring for Alan and she does not want to take the chance of ending up in the same posi-tion. The geneticist whom she saw 3 years earlier gave her a 1 in 2 risk of carrying the same gene fault as her mother, and so a 1 in 8 chance that a pregnancy would result in the birth of a boy with problems similar to Alan. As there is no specific test for the condition, Jane would like to have fetal sexing performed with a view to terminating a male pregnancy.

How is the fetal sexing performed?

As there is a 1 in 2 chance that the outcome of the test will be termination of pregnancy, the majority of women requesting fetal sexing choose CVS as it is performed earlier in the pregnancy. DNA is extracted from the chorionic villi and tested (Fig. 6.8) to ensure that there is no maternal contamina-tion of the sample. At the same time a PCR is per-

BOX 6.5 FETAL CHROMOSOME ANALYSIS

May be carried out when:

◆ one parent has been shown to carry a balanced chromosome rearrangement
◆ an increased trisomy risk has been identified
◆ there is a suggestion from ultrasound scanning that a chromosome abnormality may be present (e.g. holoprosencephaly, polydactyly and cardiac defects are associated with trisomy 13)
◆ CVS, amniocentesis or fetal blood sampling is being undertaken for another reason (e.g. prenatal DNA diagnosis etc.)
◆ there is significant maternal anxiety

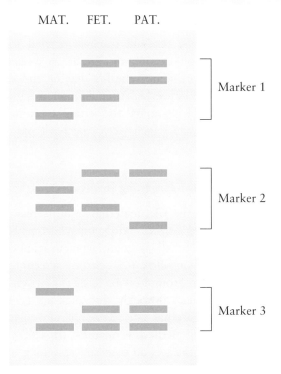

Fig. 6.8 DNA testing of CVS to exclude maternal contamination. Hypothetical result obtained using three 'CA' repeat markers (see Chapter 4, Box 4.2). The fetus (middle lane) inherits one allele from each parent (maternal on the left, paternal on the right).

formed using primers which amplify Y chromosome specific DNA sequences (Fig. 6.10). If the fetus is male, there is amplification of the DNA and a Y chromosome specific band is seen on the gel. The test result is usually available within 48 h.

Fetal chromosomes can be analysed by looking at cells obtained at chorionic villus sampling, amniocentesis or fetal blood sampling. In general the quality of the preparations from chorionic villi tends to be poorer and amniocentesis is the investigation of choice in the majority of couples carrying balanced translocations. The incidence of chromosomal mosaicism in CVS which is subsequently shown to be of no clinical significance can raise patient anxiety, and a warning about this potential complication should be built into the pre-CVS counselling session.

The CVS is also cultured for confirmatory karyotyping.

What was the result of the prenatal test?

The CVS was performed without difficulty and DNA testing showed the fetus to be female. A week later, a 46,XX karyotype is reported by the cytogenetics laboratory (**Box 6.5**)and Jane continued with the pregnancy.

CASE 6.3
Balanced translocation

Family tree

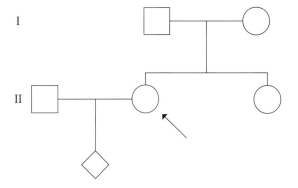

Presenting problem

Joan (II-2) is a 32-year-old psychologist who has requested prenatal testing because she is anxious that her baby may have a chromosome defect. She is 8 weeks' pregnant and is unsure which test to have.

What options are available to Joan?

Most obstetricians would discourage a woman under 35 with no family history of a chromosome abnormality from prenatal testing. If serum screening for Down syndrome (**Box 6.6**) is available, this will be discussed as an alternative. In Joan's situation, the risk of an abnormality is low but if she continues to request a diagnostic test, amniocentesis is more appropriate than CVS because of the lower associated miscarriage risk.

Joan insists on amniocentesis at 14 weeks and this is carried out without difficulty. The karyotype shows an apparently balanced translocation 46,XX,t(13;18)(q12;p11). The obstetrician checks Joan and her partner's karyotypes, both of which are normal.

What are the implications of this result?

Both amniocentesis and CVS can give unexpected karyotype results, in particular sex chromosome aneuploidies (**Box 6.7**), apparently balanced translocations (Chapter 2, Box 2.3) and ESACs (Chapter 2, Box 2.2).

When an unexpected balanced translocation is detected at amniocentesis or CVS the first step is to check both parents' karyotypes to ascertain whether the translocation is *de novo* or familial. A baby inheriting the same balanced form of a translocation present in one parent would not be expected to exhibit an abnormal phenotype as a result of this translocation. If neither parent carries a balanced translocation, then there is a risk currently estimated at about 5% that the baby may have a phenotypic abnormality, in particular mental handicap, as a *de novo* apparently balanced translocation may really be unbalanced, and therefore a cytogenetically undetectable piece of chromosome may be missing. Alternatively the translocation breakpoint may have disrupted a specific gene.

Having requested prenatal testing in order to reduce uncertainty about fetal outcome, Joan and her partner therefore have to decide whether

to continue the pregnancy given a 5% risk of abnormality.

CASE 6.4
Increased Down syndrome risk

Family tree

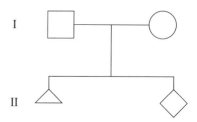

Presenting problem

Carol (I-2) is a 32-year-old teacher married to Brian, a 35-year-old accountant. She is 16 weeks into her second pregnancy, the first having ended in miscarriage at 10 weeks. After discussion with the midwife Carol has opted for serum screening for Down syndrome which has come back indicating a risk of 1 in 80.

What does serum screening involve?

In some areas of the UK, maternal serum screening for neural tube defects and Down syndrome is routinely offered to all pregnant women around 16 weeks' gestation (**Box 6.6**). Serum screening routinely picks up around 60–65% of Down syndrome pregnancies, although this pick-up rate increases with maternal age. Research into first trimester screening methods is ongoing. (**Box 6.7**). An advantage of the second trimester screening is that over 90% of open neural tube defects (spina bifida and anencephaly) will also be detected through a combination of maternal serum AFP screening and ultrasound.

Having identified the pregnancy as being of 'high risk', what options are available to Carol?

Carol has a few options. She can have a diagnostic procedure by either amniocentesis or CVS, rely on less accurate but non-invasive tests such as

BOX 6.6 BIOCHEMICAL SCREENING IN PREGNANCY

Maternal serum screening is usually performed at 16–18 weeks. It is important that the gestation of the pregnancy is assessed so that the tests can be interpreted accurately.

Neural tube defects

The first biochemical screening test to be used widely in pregnancy was measurement of maternal serum alphafetoprotein (AFP). Maternal serum AFP levels are significantly raised in the majority of pregnancies complicated by a neural tube defect (spina bifida and anencephaly). There is a considerable overlap between the upper limit of AFP concentration in normal pregnancies and the lower limit in pregnancies complicated by a neural tube defect.

Down syndrome

Most screening programmes for Down syndrome are based on two biochemical markers, maternal serum AFP and maternal serum human chorionic gonadotrophin (hCG). Some centres include a third marker, maternal serum unconjugated oestriol (uE$_3$). The levels of these markers can be combined with maternal age to give a Down syndrome risk estimate. The cut-off for a 'significantly increased risk' varies between centres but is usually taken as 1 in 250 to 1 in 280. At this risk a diagnostic test such as amniocentesis is offered. About 5% of all pregnancies will fall into this 'increased risk category', the vast majority of which will be unaffected.

Biochemical markers

◆ **alphafetoprotein** (AFP) is produced early in pregnancy by the fetal yolk sac and later by the fetal liver. It is detectable in maternal serum from about 6 weeks of pregnancy, with levels peaking at the end of the first trimester. From then until term, although the level of synthesis remains constant, maternal serum levels decrease due to the diluting effect of the increasing maternal blood volume. AFP levels are raised in several conditions including twin pregnancy, neural tube

defects and omphalocoele. Low levels of AFP indicate that the pregnancy is at increased risk of Down syndrome although the underlying mechanism is not known (Fig. 6.9a).

◆ **human chorionic gonadotrophin** (hCG) is a glycoprotein hormone secreted by the syncytiotrophoblast which appears in the maternal serum after implantation of the blastocyst. Levels rise until week 10 then fall gradually until about week 18, after which levels remain constant until term. A high serum hCG measurement is indicative of an increased Down syndrome risk (Fig. 6.9b).

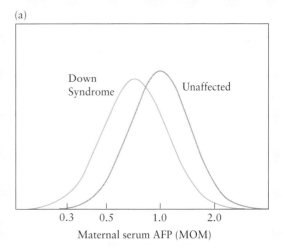

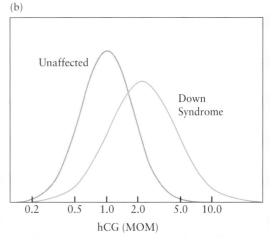

Fig. 6.9 Maternal serum AFP (a) and hCG (b) levels in Down syndrome pregnancies. MOM, multiples of the median.

BOX 6.6 BIOCHEMICAL SCREENING IN PREGNANCY (Cont.)

◆ **maternal unconjugated oestriol** (uE$_3$) is produced by fetal and placental modification of the steroid hormone oestriol which is synthesized by the syncytiotrophoblast.

Other biochemical markers such as Inhibin A are being assessed in an attempt to develop first trimester biochemical screening tests.

---

detailed ultrasound scanning, or she can opt to take no further action. Although non-invasive, second trimester ultrasound screening will only detect abnormalities associated with Down syndrome in about 50% of cases. Alternatively, amniocentesis has a small miscarriage risk and fetal karyotyping, although diagnostic, routinely involves a 3 week wait for results as the amniocytes require to be cultured. Recently it has been possible, by means of fluorescent in situ hybridization (FISH, Chapter 2,

BOX 6.7 FIRST TRIMESTER DOWN SYNDROME SCREENING

First trimester Down syndrome screening is available at present in only a few specialist centres. It is performed between 10–14 weeks' gestation.

◆ Ultrasound is used to measure fetal crown to rump length, to accurately date the pregnancy
◆ With the fetus in full profile the area of nuchal translucency is measured (this is increased in Down syndrome pregnancies)
◆ The fetal heart rate is measured (this is increased in Down syndrome pregnancies)
◆ maternal serum free hCG is measured as well as serum PAPP-A levels (increased and decreased respectively in affected pregnancies)

These criteria, in conjunction with maternal age, are then used to calculate a risk of the pregnancy being affected.

First trimester CVS can be offered as a diagnostic procedure in high risk pregnancies.

There is evidence that the pregnancies which are high risk on screening, but have normal chromosomes, have a higher risk of having a cardiac defect and therefore a detailed scan is offered later in the pregnancy.

Fig. 2.11A), to exclude or confirm a Down pregnancy on uncultured amniocytes and thus to reduce the time from amniocentesis to a result to 1 week.

After further discussion with the midwife, Carol decides that she wants to proceed to amniocentesis. However, Brian is unhappy with this course of action arguing that termination for Down syndrome is immoral.

How can this dichotomy be resolved?

Although ideally a couple should have had counselling prior to opting for serum screening, the majority opt for testing assuming that the result will be "normal". In Carol's and Brian's situation, it is important for the counsellor to facilitate communication between the couple, to help them to establish any common ground. Information should be given on the clinical aspects of Down syndrome (Chapter 2, Case 2.2) and the counsellor should ensure that both Carol and Brian understand the risk indicated by the serum screening result, which is a little less than 2%. The couple must be given sufficient time to consider their course of action – forcing either into an untenable position may jeopardize their relationship.

After discussion, Carol and Brian agree to proceed with the amniocentesis, although Brian is still unhappy about the prospect of terminating a pregnancy. The test is performed without difficulty and shows a female fetus with a karyotype of 47,XX,+21 in 1 out of 100 cells cultured. The other cells have a normal 46,XX karyotype.

What information should be given to the couple?

Trisomy 21 mosaicism at such a low level is almost certainly a culture artifact and unlikely to have any phenotypic effect on the fetus. It is important that the parents are informed of this result and the likelihood of it being a cultural artifact. At this stage, a detailed ultrasound scan can provide reassurance.

After a detailed ultrasound examination showed no evidence of fetal abnormality, the couple decided to proceed with the pregnancy.

CASE 6.5
Prenatal diagnosis for Duchenne muscular dystrophy, an X-linked disorder

Family tree

Presenting problem

Sonia (II-2) is the 25-year-old sister of 19-year-old Jimmy (II-3) who has Duchenne muscular dystrophy (DMD). Jimmy is wheelchair bound and requires artificial ventilation at night. Molecular genetic studies have shown Jimmy to carry a deletion in exon 39 of the dystrophin gene. Sonia has been tested and told that she carries the same deletion (Chapter 7, Case 7.2). Finding herself unexpectedly pregnant, she contacts the genetics department. At the same time her GP arranges an ultrasound scan which shows the pregnancy to be of approximately 9 weeks' gestation.

What are the options open to Sonia?

As this pregnancy is unplanned, Sonia may be considering termination. This option would be available to her if her doctor felt that the pregnancy

met the conditions of the 1967 Abortion Act (see **Box 6.8**). Alternatively Sonia may wish to proceed with the pregnancy either with or without prenatal testing.

Sonia and her partner decide that they can cope with a baby providing it does not have DMD and request prenatal testing.

What tests can be offered to Sonia?

As Sonia is a known carrier of an X-linked disorder (DMD), she has a 1 in 2 chance of a son being affected. The mutation in Jimmy has been characterized and therefore direct mutation analysis is possible in this pregnancy. Fetal DNA for testing can be obtained by CVS after 10 weeks. Initial tests determine fetal sex (Fig. 6.10), and mutation analysis is usually only undertaken if the

---

BOX 6.8 TERMINATION FOR FETAL ABNORMALITY IN MAINLAND BRITAIN

The 1967 Abortion Act was introduced to protect women and their doctors from prosecution under the Offences Against the Person Act (1861) when specified criteria for abortion are met. The Abortion Act was amended in 1990 by the Human Fertilization and Embryology Act which effectively removed the upper limit for gestational age as defined by the Infant Life (Preservation) Act of 1929 (28 weeks).

A pregnancy can be terminated up to 24 weeks '*if the continuation of the pregnancy would involve risk, greater than if the pregnancy were terminated, of injury to the physical or mental health of the pregnant woman or any existing children of her family*'.

A pregnancy can be terminated at any gestation if '*there is a substantial risk that if the child were born it would suffer from such physical or mental abnormalities as to be seriously handicapped*'. Alternatively if continuation of the pregnancy would result '*in grave permanent injury to the physical or mental health of the pregnant woman*' or would involve a risk to her *life* greater than if the pregnancy was terminated.

fetus is male. Prenatal female carrier status testing is not normally performed.

In Sonia's case fetal sexing showed that the fetus was male and so PCR analysis was performed to ascertain whether he carries the exon 39 deletion present in Sophia and Jimmy (Chapter 7, Case 7.2). The deletion was not detected, diagnosing the fetus as unaffected, and Sonia continued the pregnancy.

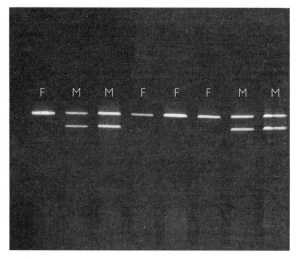

Fig. 6.10 Determination of gene by PCR. The PCR primers amplify the pseudo-autosomal boundary of X and Y chromosomes (see Fig. 7.3). The amplification of the larger PABX band serves as an internal control for failure of the male-specific PABY to amplify.

FURTHER READING

Brock DGH, Rodeck CH, Ferguson Smith MA (1992) *Prenatal Diagnosis and Screening.* Churchill Livingstone, Edinburgh.

QUESTIONS (ANSWERS ON PAGE 172)

I Amniocentesis
a has a lower risk of an ambiguous result than CVS.
b should be offered to the 30-year-old mother of a child with cleft palate.
c can be performed trans-cervically or trans-abdominally.
d has an associated miscarriage rate of 0.5–1.5%.
e is carried out under ultrasound guidance.

2 Ultrasound scanning
a may detect anencephaly at 13 weeks.
b may occasionally cause renal abnormalities.
c can be used to detect skeletal dysplasias.
d can produce an accurate estimation of gestation.
e can be used to monitor fetal growth.

3 Chorionic villus sampling is the investigation of choice for women with
a small familial translocations.
b a son with a dystrophin deletion.
c a raised serum AFP.
d myotonic dystrophy.
e a CFTR mutation in themselves and their partner.

4 A raised maternal serum AFP is associated with the following fetal malformations
a anencephaly
b Down syndrome
c exomphalos
d spina bifida
e cleft palate.

7

Carrier Testing and X-linked Inheritance

LEARNING OBJECTIVES

After studying this chapter, the reader should understand:

● the principles of X-linked inheritance and how to assess carrier risk based on Mendelian rules

● the limitations to biochemical testing for heterozygous carriers of X-linked diseases

● some of the ways in which the phenomenon of X-inactivation can aid or hinder the detection of carrier women

INTRODUCTION

One absolute rule distinguishes X-linked from autosomal inheritance: there can be no male to male transmission (since a father passes a Y but no X to his sons; Fig. 7.1). Conversely, if a male affected with an X-linked recessive disease (such as haemophilia) reproduces, *all* his daughters will be carriers (such women do not need carrier testing to determine their status!).

Because of this simple law of inheritance, when a boy with an X-linked disease is diagnosed, attention must focus on his mother's side of the family. His mother, however, may or may not be a carrier, depending on whether the affected child is the result of a new mutation. The probability of this varies from one disorder to another.

The greater part of carrier testing concerns the identification of female carriers of X-linked recessive diseases. This is because such women are at 25% risk of having an affected child each time they reproduce. Also, many such women may not

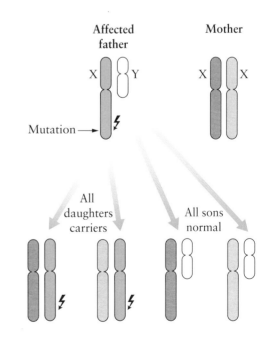

Fig. 7.1 X-linked inheritance.

suspect that they are carriers, since the recessive mutation may be passed silently for several generations through the female germ-line. Although the advent of molecular genetics has simplified carrier testing in some circumstances, there are still many cases where it is not possible to be certain about an individual's carrier risk. As much information as possible should be taken into account when attempting to determine this risk. Examples of such methods, some very indirect, are given below.

With a few exceptions (Chapter 5), carrier testing for autosomal recessive diseases is less important, since carriers of recessive autosomal mutations are only at risk of having affected children if their partner is also a carrier. For rare diseases for which the carrier frequency in the general population is low, this risk is small. The exceptions to this general principle include diseases which are common in particular populations (such as thalassaemia in Greek Cypriots, or Tay–Sachs disease in Ashkenazi Jews) and ethnic groups in which consanguineous matings are common.

CASE 7.1
Severe haemophilia A

Family tree

Presenting problem

George (II-1), aged 18 months, has been diagnosed as having severe haemophilia. He had presented with painful bilateral swelling of both knee joints, without an apparent history of trauma. The joint swellings were the result of spontaneous bleeding into the joints. Investigations showed his coagulation factor VIII level to be less than 0.5% of normal. His mother's sister Ruth (I-3) then requested investigations to determine her carrier status.

What is haemophilia?

Haemophilia presents clinically as a spontaneous bleeding disorder. It occurs due to deficiency in one of two coagulation factors, factor VIII (F8C) or factor IX (F9C). It is important to make an accurate haematological diagnosis of haemophilia A (as in this case) or haemophilia B (factor IX deficiency), which are clinically indistinguishable. Both conditions are X-linked recessives, but they result from mutations in different genes, located in chromosomal bands Xq28 (*F8C*) and Xq27 (*F9C*). Haemophilia is thus an example of a disease showing locus heterogeneity. Haemophilia A and B are also disorders which show allelic heterogeneity (see Chapters 2 and 4).

What possibilities for carrier testing in Ruth could be considered?

Factor VIII levels

Before the advent of molecular genetics, the only test which could be offered in this situation would be measurement of Ruth's own coagulation factor levels; carriers have on average lower levels of factor VIII than normal women, because only one of their two X chromosomes has a functional gene on it. Measurement of factor VIII levels for carrier detection can be complicated to interpret, due to X inactivation. Since males and females require the same dose of X-specific gene products (such as dystrophin or factor VIIIc) but have different numbers of X chromosomes, a mechanism must exist for dosage compensation, for at least most genes on the X chromosome. This is in fact achieved by shutting down almost the whole of one X chromosome in any XX cell, a process known as X inactivation (**Box 7.1**). The great majority, though not all, genes on the X are subject to X inactivation (**Box 7.2**).

Because of the random and clonal nature of X-inactivation, a female carrier of an X-linked recessive disorder has a mixture of cells expressing the normal gene and cells expressing the mutated gene in question. These two populations may be unevenly distributed, with one or the other predominating in an individual tissue or organ, either as a result of chance alone, or as a result of selection. This vari-

BOX 7.1 X INACTIVATION

The exact mechanism by which cells randomly assign one or other X chromosome for inactivation is incompletely understood. However, it appears that the process of inactivation spreads from an X inactivation centre on Xq. One gene near the X inactivation centre, named *XIST*, has the unusual property of being expressed from the inactive but not the active X. The product of the *XIST* gene is believed to be important for maintaining the silenced state of the rest of the chromosome from which it is being expressed.

Figure 7.2 is a schematic of X inactivation in the female embryo. Only nuclei of cells are shown for clarity. The maternally derived X is light blue, the paternal dark blue. Both X chromosomes are active in the very early embryo. The decision of which X to inactivate is taken *randomly and independently* in each of perhaps a few hundred cells comprising the

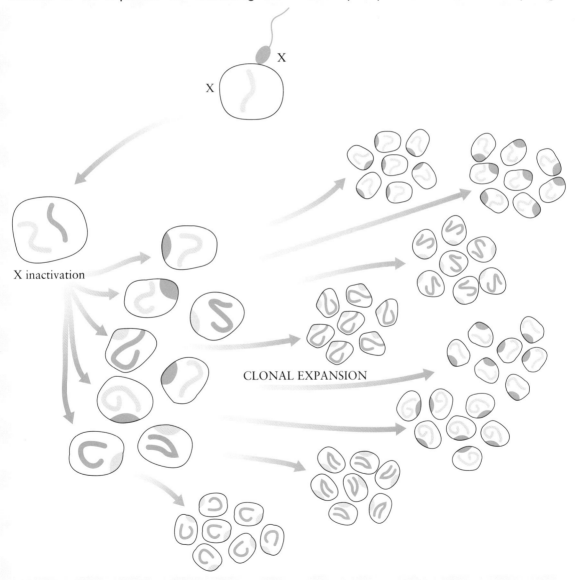

Fig. 7.2 X inactivation in the female embryo.

BOX 7.1 X INACTIVATION (Cont.)

early embryo. Some cells therefore express genes from the maternal X while others express from the paternal X. (The inactivated X is shown as a condensed mass of the corresponding colour at the side of the nucleus.) Once each of these precursor cells has made its choice, the inactivated state of that X chromosome is perpetuated in all its progeny. Thus each precursor cell gives rise to a *clone*

of cells, within which all cells have the same active X. This is the meaning of the phrase *random and clonal* applied to X inactivation. The mature female individual may be considered a 'mosaic' of different clones, each derived from one of the precursor cells, and falling into two classes according to which X is active in that clone.

BOX 7.2 PSEUDOAUTOSOMAL REGION

A few genes on the X chromosome escape inactivation; that is they are expressed from both alleles in females. This group includes genes within the pseudoautosomal region of the X, at the tip of Xp. This is a region of homology between the X and Y chromosome, within which crossing over occurs between X and Y during meiosis in males. Y specific and X specific genes lie outside the pseudoautosomal region and hence are not exchanged between X and Y during meiosis. Most importantly, one such Y specific gene is the gene which determines male sex, *SRY*. It is important that this gene remains on the Y chromosome and it therefore lies outside the pseudoautosomal region.

Figure 7.3 shows the small region at the tip of the X and Y chromosomes within which crossing over occurs (indicated by the cross) during male meiosis. Most of the sequences on the X (dark blue) and on the much smaller Y chromosome (light blue) do not show homology, but the **pseudoautosomal region** is a region in common between X and Y (medium blue, bracketed). *PABX, PABY* are the pseudoautosomal boundaries on X and Y respectively. Note that the sex-determining gene *SRY*, which dictates testis formation during embryonic

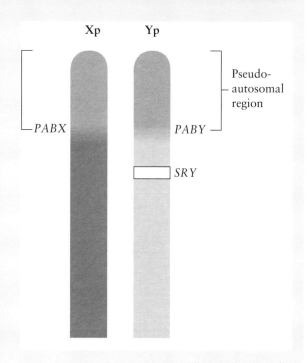

Fig. 7.3 Pseudoautosomal region of X and Y chromosomes.

development, is in the Y specific region below *PABY*, since it is unique to the Y and must not be crossed over onto the X.

ability complicates biochemical testing for X-linked diseases. A female carrier of a severe allele of haemophilia A (one resulting in <1% factor VIIIc activity in affected males) would be expected to have 50% of the normal plasma factor VIIIc activity.

However, the distribution of X inactivation in the factor VIII producing cells in the liver will play a major role in determining whether this is in fact the case or not. A slight skewing in favour of inactivation of the mutated X will give a factor VIII level within the normal range. Conversely, skewing in the opposite direction will give values <50%, though only very occasionally will this skewing be extreme enough to cause a noticeable coagulation problem. The practical consequence of this is that although a low VIIIc level may be a useful indication that a woman is a carrier, a value in the normal range gives little reassurance. The VIIIc level may sometimes be used to calculate a conditional probability for incorporation into a Bayesian calculation (Case 7.3).

Molecular analysis

One unusual type of mutation has been found to be common as a cause of severe haemophilia A, and since it can easily be tested for in carriers, it is important to know whether this particular mutation causes George's haemophilia. The nature of this mutation is illustrated in Fig. 7.4.

About half of severe cases of haemophilia A result from a large inversion of part of chromosome band Xq28. This inversion bisects the *F8C* gene, destroying its function. At the ends of the inverted segment, new restriction fragments are generated, which can be detected by Southern blotting. This offers a simple carrier test, as shown in Fig. 7.5.

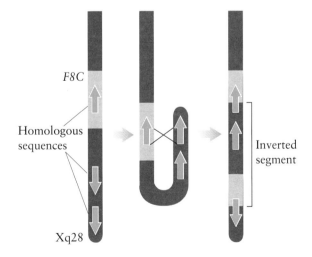

Fig. 7.4 Schematic illustration of the origin of a common mutation causing haemophilia A. The *F8C* gene is light grey. It contains DNA sequences (blue arrow) which are also present (in opposite orientation) more distally on the X chromosome. Recombination between these repeats results in inversion of the segment between them, thus bisecting the *F8C* gene.

What did molecular testing show in this family?

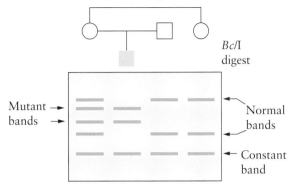

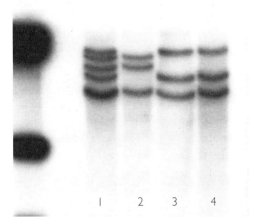

Fig. 7.5 Results of carrier test for haemophilia A. (Figure supplied by Dr L Strain)

Figure 7.5 shows the results of the molecular testing. In lane 2, the two abnormal fragments detected by the *F8C* probe (inverted X chromosome in the affected boy) are easily distinguishable in size from the two normal fragments seen in his father (lane 3). The probe also detects a constant band at the bottom of the gel, which is not involved in the inversion, on all X chromosomes. The patient's mother (lane 1) has both the two normal and two abnormal fragments, showing her to be a carrier. (In fact, for this inversion mutation, virtually *all* mothers of affected boys seem to be carriers. The new inversion mutation only occurs during spermatogenesis, so that the new mutation offspring are carrier females, not affected boys.) The mother's sister Ruth (lane 4) is clearly not carrying the abnormal DNA fragments and is therefore not a haemophilia carrier. No further tests would be needed in this situation.

Duchenne muscular dystrophy

Family tree

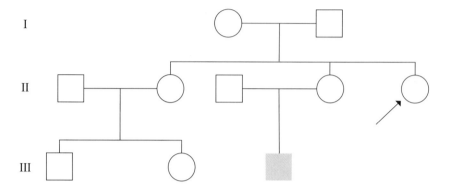

Presenting problem

Emma (II-5) has just got married. Six months ago, her 2½-year-old nephew Thomas (III-3) was referred to a paediatrician because of worries about his development. At that time, he was only just starting to walk. The paediatrician found that he had poor motor skills and noticed swelling of his calf muscles. The serum levels of the muscle enzyme creatine kinase (CK) were found to be grossly elevated, suggesting a diagnosis of muscular dystrophy, and a muscle biopsy was then performed. This showed evidence of muscle fibre death and regeneration, and irregularity of fibre size. Immunohistochemical staining for the muscle protein dystrophin showed absence of the normal pattern of dystrophin beneath the muscle fibre membrane (Fig. 7.6). On the basis of all these findings, Thomas was diagnosed as having Duchenne muscular dystrophy (DMD). Since Duchenne muscular dystrophy is an X-linked disorder, Emma has become very anxious, after talking to Thomas's mother, that she may be a carrier of DMD.

What is Duchenne muscular dystrophy?

Duchenne mucular dystrophy is a muscular degenerative disorder in which affected boys are often late in learning to walk and then become progressively weaker until they require a wheelchair.

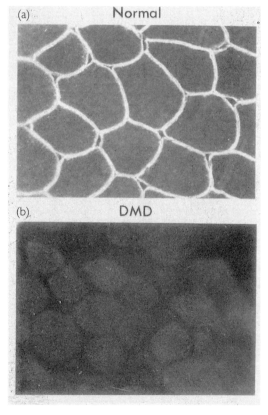

Fig. 7.6 Immunohistochemical staining of muscle fibres with dystrophin antibody. Note normal peripheral staining pattern in healthy muscle (a) and total lack of staining in muscle fibres from a Duchenne muscular dystrophy patient (b). (Figure supplied by Dr C. Bushby.)

Death due to respiratory muscle failure often occurs in their late teens. The disease is associated with very high levels of serum creatine kinase, released by damaged muscles. The disease is due to mutation in the dystrophin gene at Xp21.1. About 70% of boys with DMD have part or all of the very large (2.2 million bp) dystrophin gene missing. These deletions may be demonstrated either by PCR or Southern blotting

Is Emma a carrier for DMD?

In an isolated case of Duchenne muscular dystrophy, the situation is always initially unclear. In contrast to haemophilia, new mutations are common, and there is only a two-thirds chance of the mother of the affected boy being a carrier. Molecular genetic testing of an affected male is the first step in attempting to advise women who are at risk of being carriers. Thomas was shown to have a large deletion extending from exon 39 to beyond the 3' end of the dystrophin gene.

Analysis of CA microsatellite polymorphisms within the dystrophin gene then provided a rapid and definitive answer on the question of his aunt's

carrier status. The results for one such marker are shown in Fig. 7.7, in a form similar to their electrophoretic appearance. Three alleles of the polymorphism are distinguishable, as indicated to the right. (Note the 'shadow' bands beneath the main band which dictate care in interpretation of the pattern. See Fig. 4.4b in Chapter 4 for a photograph of such a polymorphism.)

This particular polymorphic marker does not amplify at all in the affected boy, confirming that it lies within the deleted region (lane 5). His mother, in contrast, is heterozygous for the marker (lane 4). Since her two allelic copies of the dystrophin gene are clearly distinguishable, neither can carry a deletion encompassing this marker. The test is a clear indicator of a new mutation in Thomas, and demonstrates that his mother is not a carrier. It is theoretically still possible that she could be a gonadal mosaic (Chapter 8). However, in this case she would have inherited undeleted dystrophin genes from both parents, and the mutation would have occurred during her own embryonic development. There would therefore be no increased risk of the grandmother I-2, or of the sister Emma (II-5, lane 7) being carriers. Note that

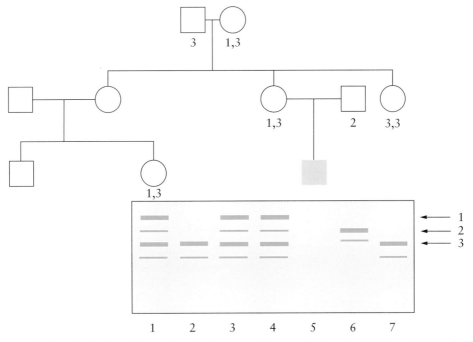

Fig. 7.7 Results of testing the family with a marker for the dystrophin gene. This marker is deleted in the affected boy.

this test performed on the sister II-5 alone, without analysis of II-3, would not have resolved the former's status. The banding pattern from the PCR as in lane 7 cannot distinguish a 3,3 homozygote from a 3,- deletion carrier. However, with the results shown for the whole family, the test is unequivocal.

What other methods are useful for carrier detection in DMD?

Creatinine kinase levels

As already mentioned, affected boys have very high levels of creatine kinase (CK) and although measurement of CK in carrier females can be helpful, as with factor VIII deficiency, X inactivation can cause problems in interpretation. Many DMD carriers have elevated serum CK levels. However, many do not; the reason is presumably that there is a skewing of X inactivation in favour of inactivating the mutated X. This skewing may not need to be very extreme to protect almost all muscle fibres, since each is multinucleate and can perhaps remain healthy even if most of its nuclei have inactivated the normal X. In a population of obligate DMD carriers, the resulting distribution of CK levels is a very broad bell-shaped curve, overlapping extensively with the narrower distribution seen in normal women (Fig. 7.8). As for haemophilia, a clearly abnormal CK value may be a valuable indicator of carrier status, but a result

nearer to normal can only be used to derive a *relative* risk for use in a Bayesian calculation.

Molecular analysis

When no deletion or other mutation can be identified in an individual affected with DMD, carrier testing of females in the family is likely to depend on linkage methods (see Chapter 4). Even in a family in which a deletion is present, simple DNA methods may not resolve females' carrier status. This is because the presence of the other normal dystrophin gene prevents simple deletion detection. PCR of the deleted area in an affected boy produces no PCR product. However, in a carrier female the normal gene will amplify and although in theory the PCR product should be half the quantity seen in a normal female, where both genes will amplify, in practice it is difficult to distinguish between a carrier and a non-carrier female. Even Southern blotting with intragenic probes, which can also demonstrate a deletion, through bands missing in affected males, suffers from a similar limitation; detection of the half intensity bands in a carrier female is technically demanding and not to be relied upon in routine practice (Fig. 7.9).

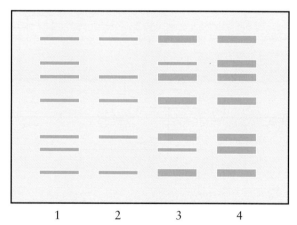

Fig. 7.9 Hypothetical Southern blot patterns detected by a dystrophin cDNA probe in a normal male (lane 1), an affected boy with an intragenic deletion (note two missing bands, lane 2) and in a female carrier of the same deletion (lane 3). DNA fragments derived from the X should be of double the intensity in females compared with males, and a deletion carrier might therefore be detectable by the diminished intensity of the bands compared to a normal female (case 4) corresponding to those deleted in the affected member of the family.

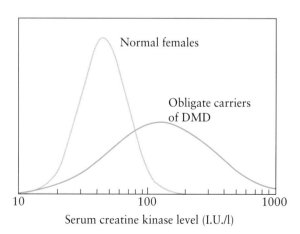

Fig. 7.8 Distribution of CK levels between normal and carrier population.

Only if a Southern blot band of altered size can be demonstrated (as for the haemophilia A inversion) is carrier detection by this method reliable. Since the deletions in DMD are usually very large, these altered junction fragments generally require pulsed-field gel electrophoresis (PFGE), a technique capable of separating extremely large DNA fragments, for their demonstration. PFGE is again a technically demanding method which requires special apparatus and sample preparation.

If a DNA probe can be identified which lies wholly within the deleted region, then fluorescent *in situ* hybridization (FISH) is applicable to carrier detection. FISH involves labelling the actual chromosome on a metaphase spread with the probe (Chapter 2, Box 2.17). If both X chromosomes in a female family member show clear hybridization signals, using a probe which is wholly deleted in the affected individual, then she is not a carrier of the deletion. If she is a carrier, then the probe will show a signal on only one X chromosome, the other X chromosome carrying the deletion.

CASE 7.3
Bayesian risk calculations

Family tree

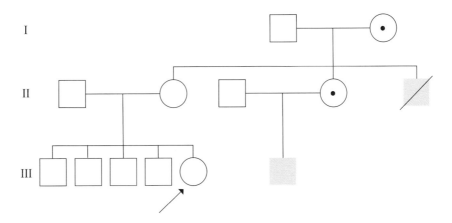

Presenting problem

Hilary, aged 18 (III-5), has been referred for genetic advice because her cousin Paul (III-6) has, and uncle Benjamin (II-5) had, Duchenne muscular dystrophy (DMD).

What is Hilary's carrier risk?

Paul's mother (II-4) is an obligate carrier of DMD as she has an affected son and brother. Her mother (I-2) is also an obligate carrier, as she has passed a DMD mutation to at least two of her offspring II-4 and II-5. Thus, the chance of Hilary's mother II-2 being a carrier should therefore be 1 in 2, and of Hilary herself being a carrier half this (1 in 4). These are Mendelian risks, which have been arrived at based solely on Hilary's position in the pedigree relative to an individual of known status (in this case I-2).

Despite this apparently logical process, common sense tells us that since Hilary's mother II-2 had four unaffected and no affected sons, she must be more likely to be a non-carrier than a carrier. It is possible to take this kind of 'hindsight' information into account, using a Bayesian calculation to arrive at a revised carrier risk. The method, for this simple example, is as follows:

For II-2 there are two mutually exclusive possibilities; she is either a carrier (C) or not a carrier (NC). The *prior* (or Mendelian) probability of each of these is, as mentioned above, 1 in 2.

For each of these two mutually exclusive scenarios, what is the probability of the observed fact, that II-2 had four normal and no affected sons?

- If she were a carrier (C), 1 in 2 of her sons would be expected to be unaffected, therefore the probability of having four sons who are unaffected is $\frac{1}{2} \times \frac{1}{2} \times \frac{1}{2} \times \frac{1}{2} = \frac{1}{16}$.
- If she were a non-carrier (NC), all of her sons would be expected to be unaffected, therefore the probability of all her sons being unaffected is 1.

These two probabilities are *conditional* probabilities. They are the chances of a known set of events having happened under two different, mutually exclusive assumptions.

By multiplying together, for each mutually exclusive path, the prior and conditional probabilities, a *joint* probability is obtained, describing how likely that combination of events would be to happen. This can be tabulated:

	C	NC
Prior probability	½	½
Conditional probability of four normal sons	⅟₁₆	1
Joint probability	⅟₃₂	½

Finally, since all other outcomes (those involving affected offspring for II-2) have been excluded using the benefit of hindsight, the two paths indicated are the only possible ones. Thus the sum of the two paths equals the total possible outcome.

The *posterior* probabilities of each of the two outcomes are therefore obtained by expressing each of the joint probabilities as a proportion of their sum.

	C	NC
Posterior probability	$\frac{1/32}{1/32 + 1/2} = \frac{1}{17}$	$\frac{1/2}{1/32 + 1/2} = \frac{16}{17}$

The posterior probability of II-2 being a carrier is therefore only ⅟₁₇, and of her daughter Hilary (III-5) being a carrier only ⅟₃₄, a long way from the gloomier estimate of ¼ from Mendelian considerations alone.

Much more complex examples can be handled

in a similar way, and conditional probabilities derived from DNA linkage or from serum creatine kinase levels (see below) can also be incorporated into the calculation. Where possible, one hopes to avoid the need for complex risk calculations by being able to test directly for the mutation, but as discussed above, this is still not always possible in DMD.

CASE 7.4
Pyruvate dehydrogenase deficiency

Family tree

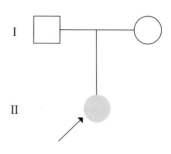

Presenting problem

Margaret (II-1) was born at term and appeared developmentally normal for the first few months of life. During her second year, however, she failed to progress, and was not walking at 18 months. During two episodes of respiratory infection, she became very weak and would not feed. When she was seen by a paediatrician at the age of 2, she showed delayed development in all areas, and was a floppy child with very poor motor skills. She was further investigated at the age of 2½, by which time she was walking with an unsteady, broad-based gait. Her blood biochemistry showed a raised level of lactate, and subsequent measurement of CSF lactate showed it too to be raised. To investigate the possible diagnosis of pyruvate dehydrogenase (PDH) deficiency, a skin biopsy was performed to measure the levels of the enzyme This gave a result within the normal range. This result, however, does not absolutely exclude the diagnosis, and when a second skin biopsy was done the following year, the PDH level was found to be reduced below the normal range, confirming a diagnosis of PDH deficiency.

What is PDH and why did the first test give a false negative result?

PDH is a multi-subunit enzyme. The E1α subunit is encoded by a gene on the X chromosome. Pyruvate dehydrogenase deficiency may cause mental handicap, structural brain abnormalities, and lactic acidosis in girls who are carriers for a defect in the X-linked E1α gene. As in this case, the enzyme deficiency may be demonstrable by enzyme assay on fibroblasts cultured from a skin biopsy. However, the clonal nature of X inactivation has a complicating effect on interpretation of the results of such a test. If (as is often the case) the skin biopsy is small, there is a good chance that most of the fibroblasts cultured will be clonally derived from one or a very few precursor cells. There is thus quite likely to be strongly skewed X inactivation simply as a result of the small sample size. If the girl in question has an E1α mutation, but in the biopsy all the cells have inactivated the mutated X chromosome, then the measured enzyme level will be completely normal. This means that the diagnosis of PDH deficiency is impossible to exclude absolutely in this way.

Can X-inactivation be helpful in diagnosing carrier status?

Clonal inactivation

As described above, the clonal inheritance of X-inactivation patterns can hinder diagnostic testing. However, in some other disorders, it may sometimes be exploited for carrier detection.

For example, in the X-linked recessive disorder, mucopolysaccharidosis type II (Hunter syndrome), the enzyme iduronidate sulphate sulphatase (IDS) is deficient. Female carriers cannot reliably be detected by simply measuring their 50% serum enzyme levels, since there is too much overlap between the normal and heterozygote levels to allow discrimination. However, individual clonal populations of cells in such individuals should have inactivated either the normal or the mutated X chromosome. This should give clones with either zero or normal enzyme levels, respectively. Heterozygotes should therefore be detectable if clonal cell populations could be identified and analysed, to demonstrate the two classes of clone. The principle of this is shown in Fig. 7.10.

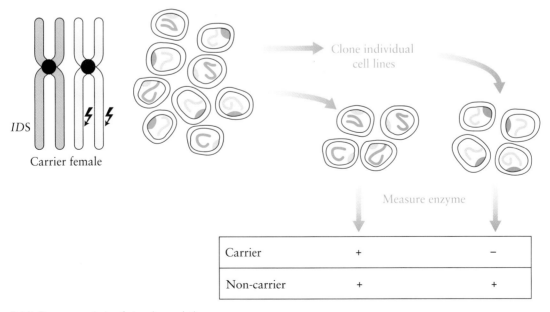

Fig. 7.10 Enzyme analysis of clonal population.

One such source of material is individual hair root bulbs. These can be pulled from suspected carriers and the enzyme level in each measured. Though hair root bulbs are not truly clonal, each does derive from a very small number of cells, so that the bimodal distribution of enzyme levels is usually demonstrable in carriers.

Skewed X inactivation

A related phenomenon occurs when the product of an X-linked gene is essential for the survival of the cell. An example of this seems to be the interleukin 2 receptor γ chain, the product of the gene responsible for X-linked recessive severe combined immune deficiency (X-SCID). A female carrier would be expected to start out as a random mosaic of cells, which have inactivated either the normal X or the one carrying the X-SCID mutation.

However, the X-SCID gene product seems to be important for T lymphocyte survival, so that lymphocyte precursors which have inactivated the normal X are selected against. This leaves a population of cells derived entirely from cells which have inactivated the abnormal X. Detection of this strongly skewed X inactivation ratio by molecular techniques is possible and may be a valuable indicator of a woman's carrier status (Fig. 7.11).

FURTHER READING

Young ID (1991) *Introduction to Risk Calculation in Genetic Counselling*. Oxford Medical Publications, Oxford.

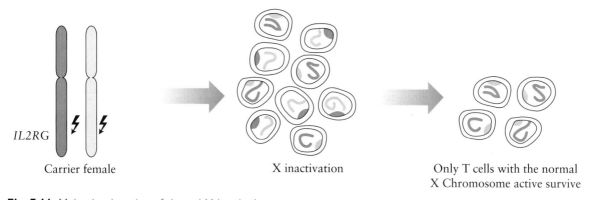

IL2RG

Carrier female   X inactivation   Only T cells with the normal
                                                               X Chromosome active survive

Fig. 7.11 Molecular detection of skewed X inactivation.

QUESTIONS (ANSWERS ON PAGE 172)

1 In an X-linked recessive disease
  a Affected boys always inherit their mutation from a carrier mother.
  b All daughters of carrier females are themselves carriers.
  c The risk of a son of an affected male being affected is zero.
  d The majority of cases will be new mutations.
  e Only males are affected.

2 The following are true of haemophilia
  a Shows allelic heterogeneity.
  b Shows locus heterogeneity.
  c The factor VIII gene inversion mutation causes mild haemophilia.
  d Only fathers transmit the inversion mutation to their offspring.
  e Shows linkage to colour blindness.

3 The following are true of Duchenne muscular dystrophy
  a One-third of isolated cases are new mutations.
  b Mutations in the same gene also cause the milder disease Becker muscular dystrophy.

  c Carriers are usually asymptomatic.
  d Carriers are often detectable using fluorescent *in situ* hybridization.
  e In diagnosis by linkage, there is an appreciable risk of error due to recombination even when using intragenic polymorphisms.

4 The following are true of X inactivation
  a Involves methylation of the inactivated chromosome.
  b Is reversed during oogenesis.
  c Spreads from the pseudoautosomal region of the X.
  d Occurs in 47,XXY males.
  e Occurs in 45,X females.

5 Which of the following may result in apparent skewing of the pattern of X inactivation?
  a Chance.
  b Selection against an X-linked mutation.
  c An X-autosome translocation.
  d A Robertsonian translocation.
  e Carrier state for haemophilia.

8

Unusual Inheritance Patterns

LEARNING OBJECTIVES

After studying this chapter, the reader should understand:

- the properties of unstable DNA or dynamic mutations, and the way in which they can lead to anomalous inheritance, either generation skipping (Fragile X syndrome) or the phenomenon of anticipation
- the general principles of maternal inheritance, and the way in which mitochondrial pathology is inherited
- the limitations of cytogenetics in detecting subtle chromosome rearrangements, and under-

stand how such rearrangements can give rise to unusual inheritance patterns
- that the paternal and maternal genetic contributions to our diploid genomes are not equivalent; know that differently imprinted parental alleles may be differently expressed, and understand the consequences of aberrant imprinting
- the existence of gonadal mosaicism and its effect upon recurrence risks for some genetic diseases.

INTRODUCTION

The cases in this chapter serve to illustrate some atypical but important inheritance patterns and to allow explanation of their genetic basis. They are a somewhat diverse group of topics, linked mainly by the fact that in each case the Mendelian 'rules'

of inheritance appear to be broken. In each case, recent application of molecular genetic technology has been needed to provide the definitive proof of the nature of the pathological processes involved.

Case 8.1
Anomalous X-linked inheritance: Fragile X

Family tree

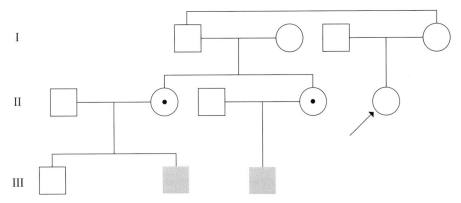

Presenting problem

Louise was referred on account of a history of mental handicap in two male relatives (III-2, III-3). One of the boys (III-2), aged 3, had recently been referred to a paediatrician due to poor speech and hyperactive behaviour. He was still not toilet trained and would not respond even to the simplest instructions from his parents. His parents complained that he would not play with anything for longer than a few seconds before moving on to something else. On physical examination little was apparent other than a large head circumference (97th centile). On the basis of the boy's clinical features and the family history, the paediatrician had suspected the diagnosis of Fragile X syndrome. A blood sample was sent for DNA analysis (see below), confirming the diagnosis. The diagnosis was then also confirmed in his cousin (III-3).

What is Fragile X syndrome?

Fragile X syndrome is known to be an X-linked form of learning difficulty. It is due to a defective *FMR1* gene, located on the X chromosome at Xq27.3. The clinical features of boys with Fragile X syndrome are not always specific enough to allow definite clinical diagnosis in young children, although affected boys are often hyperactive, with particularly marked speech delay, have larger than average head circumference, and may have unusually long ears and a slightly coarse facial appearance. Fortunately a definitive laboratory test is available to diagnose this condition.

What is the molecular basis for Fragile X syndrome?

Fragile X syndrome was initially identified when cytogenetic studies on some mentally handicapped boys, from families in which X-linked inheritance seemed to be operating, showed an unusual **fragile site** in their X chromosome at band q27.3 (Fig. 8.1). This apparent break in the chromosome was present only in a proportion of the patients' cells, and required special folate-deficient culture

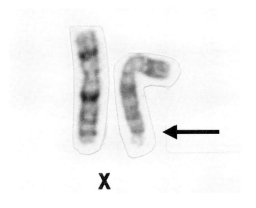

X

Fig. 8.1 Female carrier of Fragile X syndrome. Note the fragile site on one X chromosome.

conditions for its demonstration. The karyotype of an affected boy would be written 46,XY,fra(X)(q27.3). Other fragile sites have been described.

The nature of the fragile site was elucidated in 1991. This revealed that Fragile X is an unstable DNA disorder (**Box 8.1**). It results from the expansion of a CGG trinucleotide repeat situated at the 5' end of a gene at Xq27.3, named *FMR1* (fragile X mental retardation). This triplet repeat is 5–50 units long in normal individuals (i.e. is polymorphic), but hundreds or thousands of units in length in individuals with Fragile X.

It has been found that when the repeat is larger than approximately 200 triplets, the *FMR1* gene becomes methylated at its 5' end and transcriptionally inactive (see Chapter 3). The methylation pattern can be demonstrated by Southern blotting, using a methylation sensitive enzyme. The silencing of the gene and the resulting lack of FMR1 protein are responsible for Fragile X syndrome, though the exact biochemical function of the FMR1 protein in the brain still needs elucidating. Girls too can be affected by Fragile X syndrome but, in keeping with the fact that they have a normal X in addition to their full mutation-carrying X, most show milder features (in fact 50–70% of females with full mutations have IQs in the normal range).

BOX 8.1 TRINUCLEOTIDE REPEATS

(CAG)_n repeats
Some late-onset neurodegenerative diseases have in common an unusual type of mutation. The genes involved in these diseases have a $(CAG)_n$ trinucleotide repeat sequence within the coding region, which encodes a stretch of glutamine residues in the resulting proteins. Although the function of these polyglutamine tracts within the neurons is not

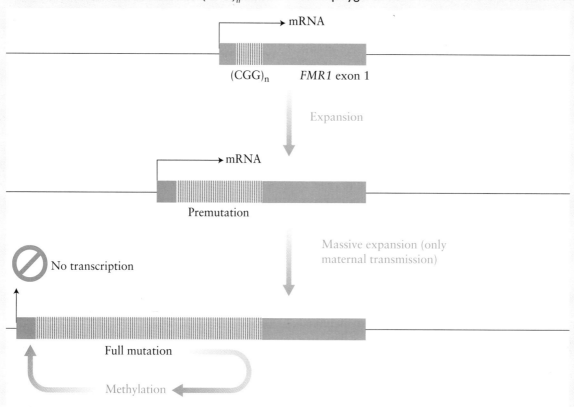

Fig. 8.2 Expansion of premutation in maternal transmission.

BOX 8.1 TRINUCLEOTIDE REPEATS (Cont.)

known, individuals affected with the diseases in question have an expanded trinucleotide repeat region, and hence a protein within their neurons which has a larger than normal polyglutamine stretch. There is also variation in size of the polyglutamine stretch within the normal population, but the ranges of sizes seen in normal and affected individuals do not generally overlap. Within the affected size range, for some of the diseases there is a correlation between the size of the expanded repeat and the age of onset or the severity of the disease; the larger the repeat, the earlier the onset.

The most important of these disorders is Huntington's disease (HD), which causes an extrapyramidal movement disorder and progressive dementia. The condition is further discussed in Chapters 4 and 5. In Fig. 8.3 can be seen the distribution of CAG repeat number in the normal and HD populations. The very fine cut-off between the normal and affected populations is striking. Like most of the other disorders in this category, HD is inherited as an autosomal dominant. In fact, it behaves as a true dominant in the Mendelian sense of the word, since individuals homozygous for the CAG repeat expansion are affected similarly to heterozygotes.

Other polyglutamine repeat disorders include: spinocerebellar atrophy type 1, SCA1; Machado–Joseph disease (spinocerebellar atrophy type 3, SCA3); dentatorubropallidoluysian degeneration (DRPLA); spinal and bulbar muscular atrophy (SBMA). All these are autosomal dominant disorders apart from SBMA, which results from an expansion within the androgen receptor gene on the X chromosome.

$(CGG)_n$ and $(CTG)_n$ repeats

These are conditions in which the triplet repeat expands to a very much greater extent than in the above disorders and, since it lies outside the coding region of the gene involved, affects gene function by other means than altering protein structure. Trinucleotide repeat disorders are sometimes

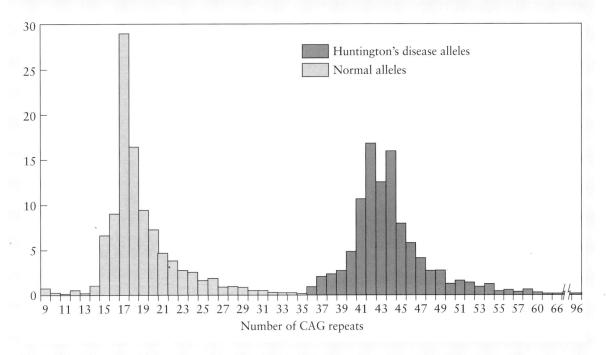

Fig. 8.3 Histogram showing the percentages of normal individuals (grey) or Huntington disease patients (blue) having CAG repeat numbers of the indicated size. (Figure supplied by Dr JP Warner and Ms L Barron.)

BOX 8.1 TRINUCLEOTIDE REPEATS (Cont.)

referred to as unstable DNA disorders. This is because the triplet repeat often changes in size when transmitted from parent to child. Instability is seen in the neurodegenerative disorders like Huntington's disease, but is much more marked in Fragile X syndrome (($CGG)_n$ repeats) and myotonic dystrophy (($CTG)_n$ repeats). For some disorders, instability is seen when a repeat above a certain size is transmitted by a parent of one sex, but not the other. In Fragile X syndrome, for example, fathers carrying expanded triplet repeats in the size range 60–200 (a so-called premutation) usually transmit the repeat to their daughters unchanged in size.

When these women pass on this repeat to their own offspring, however, it often undergoes a further dramatic expansion into the full mutation range of hundreds to thousands of triplets, which results in Fragile X syndrome.

$(CGG)_n$ repeats such as in Fragile X syndrome affect DNA methylation and produce inducible chromosomal fragile sites (Case 8.1). The expression of adjacent genes is affected. On the other hand the $(CTG)_n$ repeats found in myotonic dystrophy do correlate with the disease but their effect does not appear to be on transcription or structure of the myotonic dystrophy kinase gene product.

What information can be gained from Louise's family tree as to her risk of having an affected boy?

As Fragile X is an X-linked disorder and the mothers of the affected boys are sisters, both mothers of the affected boys must be carriers of Fragile X. If the normal rules of X-linked recessive disease are applied then Louise is at low risk of having an affected boy as she is related to these two women only through her uncle (I-1), a solicitor. Since I-1 is clearly unaffected, the X-linked mutation found in the carrier sisters II-2 and II-4 surely must have come from their mother? Unfortunately these rules break down in Fragile X syndrome and, although this is the most likely means by which the mutation has been passed through this family, it is now also known that some men in Fragile X families can have an abnormal number of the trinucleotide repeat but not be affected. These men are termed normal transmitting males.

What is the molecular basis of normal transmitting males?

The massively expanded CGG triplet array in individuals affected by Fragile X is known as a full mutation. This is to distinguish it from smaller degrees of expansion (roughly 50–200 repeats)

called premutations. Premutations do not cause methylation of the *FMR1* gene, and therefore cause no clinical problems. However, their instability and tendency to expand to full mutations means that they are important in determining the pattern of transmission within Fragile X families. Premutations may expand to full mutations when they are passed from mother to child (son or daughter).

A premutation in a male is passed down as a premutation to all his daughters. However when his daughters have children, the premutation may expand to a full mutation, causing the classical problems associated with Fragile X syndrome (see Fig. 8.2 in **Box 8.1**).

What did molecular analysis show in Louise's family?

Southern blotting is used as the main laboratory investigation in Fragile X. Part of the family tree is analysed on the gel shown in Fig. 8.4.

The key to understanding the odd inheritance of Fragile X syndrome comes from the blot pattern in the mothers of the affected boys (lanes c, e). Though each mother has, in addition to her normal X chromosome (5.1 kb fragment), a fragment of increased size, it is only slightly enlarged. However, it is large enough to be unstable on

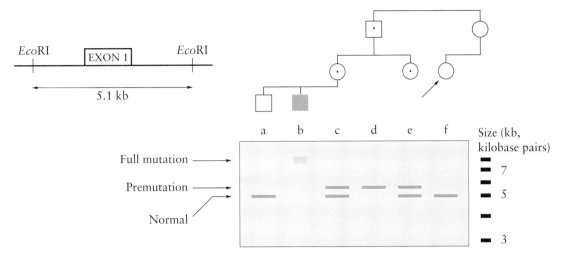

Fig. 8.4 The DNA probe used for Fragile X diagnosis detects a 5.1 kb *Eco*RI fragment from a normal X chromosome (lane a, III-1). This fragment is greatly increased in size in affected individuals because of the presence of the expanded trinucleotide repeat array (lane b, III-2). Also, because of instability of the array of thousands of triplets, there is a smear representing fragments of different sizes in individual cells, rather than a discrete band.

transmission from mother to child, resulting in the affected sons. When this so-called premutation is followed back a generation, it can be seen that it has come from the woman's own father (I-1) (lane d), who has transmitted it virtually unchanged in size, as is the rule in transmission by fathers. Because it is unmethylated (see **Box 8.1**), the premutation does not affect *FMR1* function, and thus I-1 is a so-called normal transmitting male.

Louise can no longer be reassured without investigation. Since her uncle is a normal transmitting male, her mother could also be a carrier of a premutation, or even of a 'full' mutation of the type seen in the affected boys.

Fortunately, carrier testing in Fragile X families is now a simple matter and, as seen in lane f, Southern blotting of the consultand shows her to have only normal sized fragments. She is therefore not a carrier of Fragile X syndrome.

CASE 8.2
Anticipation: myotonic dystrophy

Family tree

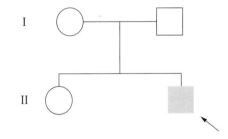

Presenting problem

Thirty-year-old Jacqueline's second pregnancy was complicated in the third trimester by polyhydramnios. There were relatively few fetal movements, but ultrasound scanning had shown no obvious structural abnormality. After a prolonged and difficult labour at 35 weeks, the baby was delivered by forceps. He was hypotonic and required resuscitation. The baby continued to have breathing difficulties, and several days of assisted ventilation were required. He fed poorly thereafter and had little facial movement. These clinical features and the obstetric history suggested the possible diagnosis of congenital myotonic dystrophy. A paediatric neurologist asked to assess the baby had this suspicion reinforced when he met Jacqueline herself. On shaking hands, he noticed her pronounced myotonia, manifested by inability to relax her grip rapidly. On questioning though, Jacqueline admitted only to mild stiffness in the mornings and no other musculoskeletal symptoms. She had wasting of the temporal muscles and clear weakness of neck flexion (sternocleidomastoid muscle weakness, often an early sign in myotonic dystrophy), as well as a mild bilateral ptosis (drooping eyelids).

Confirmation of the diagnosis of myotonic dystrophy was obtained through recording the electrical activity of Jacqueline's muscles (electromyography, EMG) and also by DNA testing (see below). EMG showed characteristic myotonic potentials.

What is myotonic dystrophy?

Myotonic dystrophy is a slowly progressive multi-system disease, in which in addition to the musculoskeletal features noted above, there may be cardiac arrhythmia or cardiomyopathy, disturbed gut motility, endocrine problems including impaired glucose tolerance and male infertility, dangerous abnormal reactions to anaesthetic drugs, and sometimes mental impairment. Congenitally affected children often have moderately severe mental handicap in addition to delay in reaching motor milestones such as sitting and walking. With rare exceptions, only affected mothers are at risk of having a congenitally affected child; this is almost never seen when the abnormal gene is transmitted by a father. Anticipation is a tendency for the disease to increase in severity with succeeding generations (e.g. Fig 8.6).

What is the molecular basis of myotonic dystrophy?

Myotonic dystrophy is another of the unstable DNA disorders (**Box 8.1**). It is inherited as an autosomal dominant (the expanded CTG repeat is present in one of the two copies of the gene, and hence transmitted with 50% probability to off-spring of affected individuals). The behaviour of

the CTG repeat gives rise to anomalous features in the inheritance of myotonic dystrophy.

The anticipation shown in families reflects a progressive expansion in size of the trinucleotide repeat, with congenitally affected infants having the largest expansions and the asymptomatic or mildly affected individuals only modest expansion in size.

What did molecular analysis show in this family?

Southern blotting of DNA from mother and child was undertaken. In both, this showed, in addition to normal sized DNA fragments, corresponding to a normal copy of the myotonic dystrophy gene on chromosome 19, an expanded, smeared fragment, diagnostic of a large expansion in the CTG trinucleotide repeat at the 3' end of the gene. Subsequent investigation of the family showed the inheritance in Fig. 8.5.

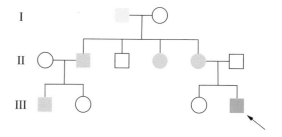

Fig. 8.5 Extended family tree after mutation analysis was performed.

Despite the presence of clear symptoms in several family members, it was not until the birth of the severely, congenitally affected baby III-4 that the diagnosis of myotonic dystrophy was made in other family members. This is commonly the case. II-2 (44 years old) had frontal balding, clear temporal and sternocleidomastoid wasting, and had complained for some years of worsening muscle stiffness. His son III-1 had grip myotonia and a positive EMG at the age of 23. Clinical features similar to those of her sister were present in II-4. All these affected individuals also had cataracts, though these had not interfered with vision. The grandfather I-1 was asymptomatic at age 67, and had no muscle weakness or myotonia on examination. However, he had dense cataracts at the posterior pole of both lenses.

CASE 8.3
Mitochondrial inheritance

Family tree

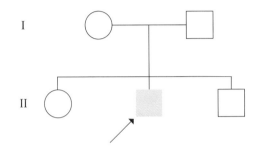

Presenting problem

Fraser, a 26-year-old man, presented to his GP with the complaint of poor eyesight. A keen cricketer, he had initially noticed problems losing sight of the ball whilst batting. On examination, large bilateral central visual field defects were demonstrated. The ophthalmologist also reported apparent elevation of the optic discs and abnormal tortuous vessels. Over the next year, the man's vision deteriorated rapidly to the point at which he could barely perceive light.

With this dramatic history and these physical findings, a diagnosis of Leber's optic atrophy (Leber's hereditary optic neuropathy, LHON) was suspected.

What is LHON?

LHON was once suspected to be an X-linked recessive condition, since it usually affects males, is familial, but is never transmitted from father to son. However, it is now appreciated that the inheritance pattern results from the maternal inheritance of mitochondria and their DNA. The male predominance is still not well understood. LHON is a disease which results from any of a number of mitochondrial DNA mutations.

What is mitochondrial DNA?

The mitochondrion is a metabolically important cytoplasmic organelle. It contains its own chromosome; a circular DNA molecule of 16 559 bp. This DNA molecule contains genes for some of the mitochondrial components, including ribosomal and transfer RNAs, some subunits of the respiratory chain complexes and some ATPase subunits (see Fig. 8.6, **Box 8.2**). Mitochondria are inherited virtually exclusively from the oocyte. A number of diseases resulting from point mutations, deletions or rearrangements of the mitochondrial genome, therefore display a characteristic maternal inheritance pattern. Mitochondrially encoded disorders cannot be paternally transmitted.

If an oocyte contains a mixture of mitochondria with normal and mutated mtDNA, both will be transmitted to daughter cells. Unlike the nuclear genome, there is no mechanism for ensuring equal segregation of the different species to progeny. Different daughter cells may contain different proportions of the mitochondrial variant. In the mature individual, correspondingly, some tissues may contain greater or lesser proportions of abnormal mitochondria. This situation, in which both normal and mutated mitochondria are contained in the same cell, is known as heteroplasmy and complicates genetic and phenotypic predictions. The level of heteroplasmy may determine the likelihood of an individual being affected (the penetrance of the disorder). Different individuals within a family may be affected to differing degrees of severity depending on the level of heteroplasmy, or may even have different clinical features because of different tissue distributions of the mutation.

There is a bewildering array of clinical presentations in mitochondrial disorders, and many different abnormalities of the mitochondrial DNA may underlie them. Many patients have myopathies with a characteristic abnormal histological pattern on muscle biopsy; red ragged fibres. The metabolic defect in the mitochondrial electron transport chain results in elevation of blood and/or CSF lactate. Some specific syndromes such as LHON have descriptive or eponymous titles.

BOX 8.2 MITOCHONDRIAL MUTATIONS

The terminology for mitochondrial mutations requires a little explanation (Fig. 8.6). Each gene on the mitochondrion has the letters MT as part of its name; for example *MTND4* is the gene encoding subunit 4 of NADH dehydrogenase (part of complex I of the mitochondrial respiratory chain). The specific mutation is indicated after the asterisk; *MTND4*11778A is a single base change at nucleotide 11 778. It causes an arginine to histidine substitution in the NADH dehydrogenase subunit 4, and thus, as with all LHON mutations, causes a respiratory chain deficit (in this case as in most LHON, a complex I defect) within the mitochondria.

◆ Myoclonic epilepsy with ragged red fibres (MERRF) – associated with a missense mutation in the gene for transfer RNA for lysine (tRNALys; *MTTK*G8344*). The A to G mutation at nucleotide 8344 accounts for 80–90% of MERRF cases.

◆ Myopathy, encephalopathy, lactic acidosis, stroke-like episodes (MELAS) – often associated with a mutation in the tRNALeu(UUR) gene; *MTTL1*G3243*.

Interestingly, this tRNALeu mutation is also found in perhaps 1% of diabetic patients, both with and without neurological features (including deafness), and sometimes with cardiomyopathy.

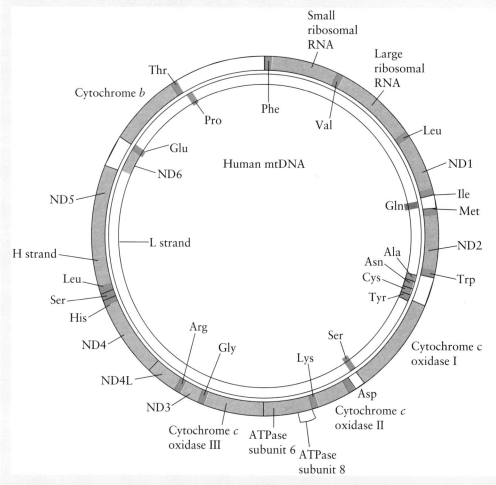

Fig. 8.6 Organization of human mitochondrial DNA (mtDNA). Protein and RNAs encoded by each of the two strands are shown separately. Transcription off the outer (H) strand of each mtDNA is clockwise and off the inner (L) strand is counterclockwise. Blue indicates tRNA gene.

What did molecular studies show in Fraser and his family?

Because LHON is a genetic disorder, DNA studies were undertaken both to confirm the diagnosis and for use in genetic counselling. Ninety per cent of patients with LHON have one of three common mutations. Analysis revealed that Fraser had the mutation *MTND4*11778A* (a point mutation at position 11 778 of the mitochondrial DNA sequence, **Box 8.2**) present in about 70% of his mitochondria, with the remainder lacking the mutation. Because of this finding, other members of the family were also tested. The mutation was present in Fraser's mother, and in his brother (age 22) and sister (age 30) (see Fig. 8.7). The propor-

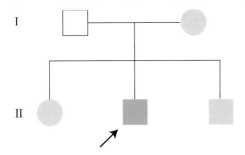

Fig. 8.7 Results of molecular studies in Fraser and his family.

tion of abnormal mitochondria was roughly estimated in each case at 40, 80 and 60%. Visual field testing in the two women was normal, but small central field defects were detected in the younger brother, who later experienced a similar rapid deterioration in visual acuity similar to that suffered by his brother.

What is the risk to the offspring of II-1?

Because a mother with a mitochondrial mutation will transmit her mitochondria to all her offspring (regardless of sex), one might predict a 100% recurrence risk for such disorders. However, the phenomenon of heteroplasmy makes the true recurrence risk very difficult to estimate. Frequently after the ascertainment of an affected individual, the mitochondrial mutation will be demonstrable in other family members, but in lower proportions than in the index case. For the reasons given above, some or many of such individuals may remain asymptomatic, making it extremely difficult to be precise about risks to offspring of women with mitochondrial mutations. The only hard and fast rule is the essentially zero risk to offspring of an affected male.

CASE 8.4
Cryptic translocations

Family tree

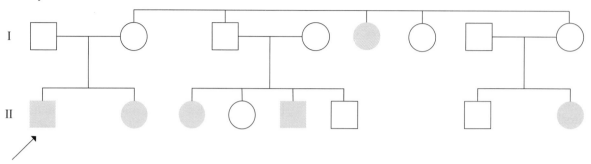

The family was referred because of several cases of unexplained mental handicap. The index case Jonathan was severely mentally handicapped and also had a number of physical malformations and facial dysmorphism. The other shaded individuals were more mildly affected but had significant learning difficulties and some facial dysmorphism. Routine karyotype analysis performed in infancy on II-1, on account of his multiple abnormalities, had shown no abnormality. A rare or unrecognized single-gene disorder had therefore been suspected in the family. However, extensive biochemical investigations of Jonathan had also been negative.

How is this disorder inherited?

Careful inspection of the family tree in fact shows that it cannot be easily fitted with any simple Mendelian inheritance pattern. Autosomal recessive inheritance is unlikely, since affected individuals have been born to three siblings with unrelated spouses (see Chapter 1). X-linked inheritance and autosomal dominant inheritance do not fit with transmission through the normal father I-3 to an affected son III-5. All the presumed 'carriers' I-2, I-3 and I-8 were completely normal.

What further investigations were performed on this family?

High resolution cytogenetics was performed on Rachel (II-8) and this showed that she had an unbalanced form of a reciprocal translocation between chromosome 2q37 and chromosome 11p15.5. (See Chapter 2 for definitions of types of translocation.) These breakpoints are almost right at the ends of the chromosomes, making the translocated segments very difficult to spot. In Rachel's mother (I-8), this translocation was present in balanced form. Rachel, however, was monosomic for the tip of chromosome 2 and trisomic for the tip of chromosome 11. This unbalanced chromosome was also present in other affected members of the family. All the parents of affected individuals (I-2, I-3 and I-8) were carriers of the translocation in balanced form.

Tiny translocations of this type may be very difficult to spot on conventional cytogenetics. Indeed, in some cases the segments translocated are so small that the translocation can only be demonstrated by fluorescent *in situ* hybridization or by analysis of DNA polymorphisms located in the chromosomal regions close to the telomeres. For this reason they are referred to a 'cryptic' translocations. Such sub-telomeric translocations have been shown to be present in a number of families with unexplained mental handicap. The way in which DNA polymorphisms can be used to demonstrate the presence of such a cryptic translocation is shown in Fig. 8.8.

Only individuals I-3, I-4 and their children are shown from the pedigree in Fig. 8.8. They are being analysed by Southern blotting, with a probe detecting a polymorphism located in the sub-telomeric region of 2q. All four of the parental alleles at the polymorphic locus are distinguish-

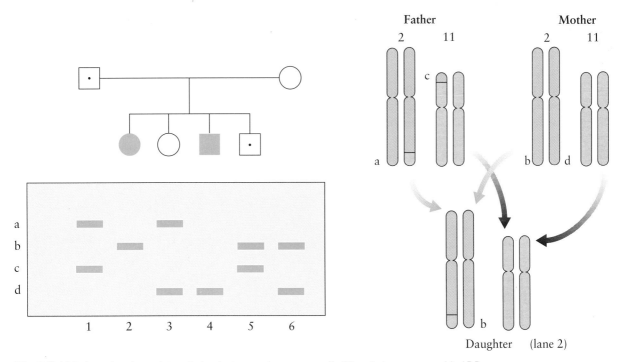

Fig. 8.8 Unbalanced reciprocal translation between chromosome 2q37 and chromosome 11p15.5.

able, and are labelled *a–d* on the Southern blot and on the chromosome diagram. Consider first the normal girl II-4 (lane 3). As expected, she has inherited one allele of the polymorphism from each parent.

In the father in this family, as shown by the chromosome sketches (chromosome 2 light blue, chromosome 11 dark blue), the allele *c* of the polymorphic marker has been translocated as part of the tiny terminal segment of chromosome 2 onto chromosome 11. The remaining der(2) is missing the subtelomeric marker, and when this der(2) is passed on to the offspring along with the father's normal chromosome 11, no paternal allele at this locus is inherited by the abnormal child. This situation is seen in lane 2; the affected girl has inherited a maternal *b* allele but no paternal allele for the 2q marker. Analysis of a subtelomeric chromosome 11p marker in the same way could also have revealed that the unbalanced offspring had inherited two paternal alleles at this site.

What about the unaffected boy? Examine lane 5. He has inherited the *c* allele carried on the der(11) from his father. He must therefore be a balanced carrier, who has inherited both the der(2) and the der(11). The best way to visualize these inheritance patterns clearly for each individual, is to draw out the four chromosomes, as for individual II-3 (lane 2).

CASE 8.5
Imprinting

Family tree

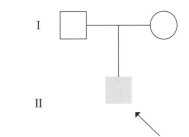

Presenting problem

James is a 5-year-old boy who has been referred to the child psychiatrist on account of behavioural problems. He had already been followed as an out-patient, since age 3, on account of developmental delay. More recently he had developed behavioural problems prompting diagnostic reassessment. He had been delivered by the breech at full-term, weighing 2.8 kg. It was immediately noted then that he was very floppy, with tendon reflexes which were difficult to elicit. These problems persisted for the first 6 months or so. During this period of infancy he fed poorly and gained weight slowly. His other main abnormality which had been noted was a very small penis and scrotum, with impalpable testes. This combination of features had suggested the diagnosis of Prader–Willi syndrome, a genetic disorder known to be associated in some cases with deletions of the short arm of chromosome 15. A chromosome analysis had therefore been ordered. This revealed a normal male karyotype, 46,XY. Further genetic investigations were now being considered.

On examination now, James was short, but markedly obese. His feet were small. Direct questioning revealed that he seemed to be constantly hungry, eating anything and everything available. He was also now rather hyperactive and had frequent temper tantrums.

What additional genetic studies can be considered?

Hyperphagia is so characteristic of Prader–Willi syndrome that despite the negative cytogenetic findings, the psychiatrist felt certain that this was the diagnosis, and requested further genetic investigations. Initially, to investigate the possibility of a deletion too small to be seen by conventional cytogenetics (a microdeletion), fluorescent *in situ* hybridization (FISH; Chapter 2, **Box 2.17**) was performed using a DNA probe derived from the region of chromosome 15q known to be critical in Prader–Willi syndrome. This showed clear fluorescent spots on both copies of chromosome 15, suggesting that no microdeletion was present. However, this still does not rule out the diagnosis of PWS.

DNA polymorphisms located near the critical region of chromosome 15 were next studied in James and his parents. Figure 8.9a shows the traces generated by PCR products of a chromosome 15

CA repeat polymorphism. Each major peak represents one allele. The two alleles present in each parent are clearly distinguishable. However, James himself appears to have two alleles, both of which are derived from his mother, instead of the expected one allele from each parent. This anomalous inheritance was also demonstrated with

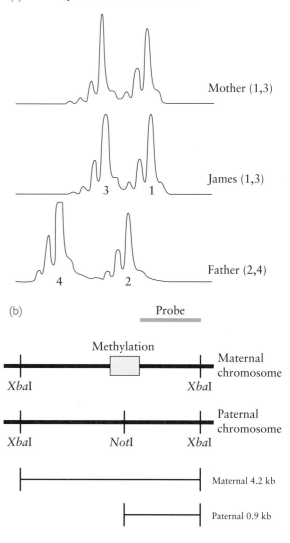

Fig. 8.9 (a) Traces derived fron an automated gel scanner of a fluorescently labelled PCR amplified CA repeat, located on chromosome 15. The PCR products are detected as peaks rather than bands on a gel; however, as for any gel, larger fragments migrate more slowly (migration direction shown by arrow), so larger fragments are to the right of the figure. Alleles are numbered 1–4, largest to smallest. The appearance ot two maternally-derived alleles but no paternal allele in James is diagonostic of uniparental disomy for chromosome 15. (b) Probe

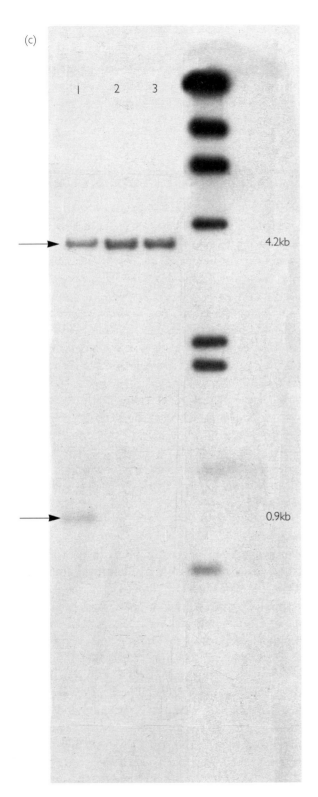

other polymorphisms on chromosome 15. This is a situation referred to as uniparental disomy. Uniparental disomy for chromosome 15 is the underlying genetic defect in about a quarter to a third of cases of PWS, and the finding confirms the diagnosis.

How might clinically indistinguishable cases of PWS result from two apparently different genetic lesions (deletion/microdeletion and uniparental disomy)?

The answer comes from consideration of the parental origin of the pathology in each case. In all cases of deletion PWS, it is the paternal chromosome 15 which is deleted. In PWS due to uniparental disomy, both chromosomes 15 are always of maternal origin. These two situations have in common the fact that a paternally derived 15q11-q13 region is missing. The clinical observations point to the fact that the maternal and paternal copies of chromosome 15q11-q13 are non-equivalent. Loss of the latter results in PWS. In contrast, loss of the maternal 15q11-q13 functions, either by a deletion on a maternal 15 or (rarely) by paternal uniparental disomy for chromosome 15, is known to cause a completely different disorder, Angelman syndrome.

What is the explanation for the maternal and paternal copies of chromosome 15q11-q13 being non-equivalent?

This situation violates the general Mendelian principle that mother and father contribute equivalent sets of autosomal genes to their offspring. Although the same genes, encoded in the same DNA sequences, are present on the paternal and maternal 15q11-q13 region, their functions are different as a result of different modifications of the DNA laid down respectively during spermatogenesis or oogenesis. This is a process called genomic imprinting (**Box 8.3**). Even in the mature individual, imprinting may be directly observable, in the form of different DNA methylation patterns of the alleles derived from mother and father. This can provide simple diagnostic tests for conditions such as PWS, as shown in Fig. 8.9b, c. Using a DNA

Fig. 8.9 (c) Sizes of fragments detected by Southern blotting using a probe for the *SNRPN* gene, in the PWS region of 15q11–13.

probe from the critical region of 15q11-q13 for Southern blotting, and cutting the target genomic DNA with a methylation-sensitive restriction enzyme (such as *Not*I), normal individuals display one methylated (maternal) and one unmethylated (paternal) allele (lane 1). If maternal uniparental disomy is present, both alleles show the maternal methylation pattern, and the fragments corresponding to the paternal hypomethylated allele are absent (lanes 2, 3). Since paternal bands on the blot will be similarly absent in the case of a paternally derived 15q deletion, this method provides a single useful unifying diagnostic test for both forms of PWS.

BOX 8.3 IMPRINTED GENES

Few genes appear to be imprinted in mammals, but there are some notable examples. The different methylation of paternal and maternal alleles during gametogenesis 'programmes' further allele specific modifications during embryonic development, with the result that there is monoallelic expression of the imprinted gene. In many tissues, the gene for insulin-like growth factor II (*IGF2*), for example, is transcribed only from the paternal allele during development, the maternal copy being silenced. Such monoallelic expression patterns may occur only in some tissues, or at particular times of development, so that imprinting provides an additional layer of gene regulation for some genes. Aberrant reactivation of the maternal *IGF2* allele has been seen in Wilms tumour, suggesting that relaxation of growth factor imprinting could contribute to tumorigenesis in some situations. In support of this mechanistic connection, some individuals with Beckwith–Wiedemann syndrome, in which fetal overgrowth is seen, have paternal uniparental disomy of chromosome 11p15, where *IGF2* resides. These patients, with two active *IGF2* alleles, are predisposed to the development of Wilms tumour.

Imprinted genes are non-randomly distributed around the chromosomes. Some imprinted 'domains' contain several imprinted genes; for example the 11p15 region containing *IGF2* also contains *H19*, *p57KIP2* and *Mash2* (all *maternally* expressed genes, in contrast to *IGF2*). There is also evidence that the insulin gene, within the same region, may be imprinted. The other side of this coin is that some whole chromosomes may have no imprinted genes at all. Uniparental disomy for chromosome 21, for example, seems to be completely without phenotypic effect.

CASE 8.6
Gonadal mosaicism

Family tree

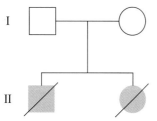

Presenting problem

Damien and Morag were referred for genetic counselling following the death of their second child in the perinatal period, from respiratory insufficiency complicating osteogenesis imperfecta. The pregnancy had been uneventful, but on delivery the baby was noted to have short deformed limbs and a narrow, asymmetrical chest. There was marked respiratory distress and the baby had been intubated at 10 minutes of age. X-rays then showed multiple fractures of the long bones and ribs and a poorly ossified skull (Fig. 8.10). These features are diagnostic of the severe, perinatally lethal form of osteogenesis imperfecta (type II). It proved difficult to maintain adequate ventilation and active support had been withdrawn after discussion of the prognosis with the parents. A skin biopsy was taken prior to the child's death.

This couple's first baby had been similarly affected and stillborn, 3 years previously. The obvious question raised was whether this family was manifesting an autosomal recessive disease.

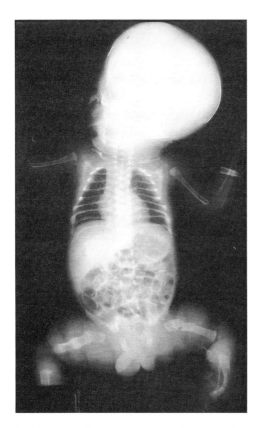

Fig. 8.10 Features of severe osteogenesis imperfecta (type IIa).

What is osteogenesis imperfecta?

Osteogenesis imperfecta is usually due to a deficiency of type I collagen, the major structural collagen of bone and tendon. There is a wide range of severity, mildly affected patients suffering recurrent fractures with fairly mild trauma during childhood, which heal well, but growing out of their fracture tendency after puberty. In one widely used clinical classification scheme, the most severely affected babies (who often have intrauterine fractures) are referred to as having type II osteogenesis imperfecta. Features commonly associated with osteogenesis imperfecta include joint laxity, blue sclerae, conductive deafness and small additional ('Wormian') bones in the skull sutures. All the clinical types of osteogenesis imperfecta result usually from mutations in either of the type I collagen genes. The triple helix of type I collagen is composed of two α_1 chains (α_1(I)) and one α_2 chain (α_2(I)). These are encoded by the COL1A1 and COL1A2 genes, on chromosomes 17q and 7q respectively. Mutations in either gene cause clinically indistinguishable phenotypes.

How is osteogenesis imperfecta inherited?

The milder types of osteogenesis imperfecta are inherited as autosomal dominants, suggesting that the responsible collagen mutation is present on only one allele of either COL1A1 or COL1A2. This has been shown by mutation analysis in several families. The transmission risk for an affected parent is of course 50%. For severe type II osteogenesis imperfecta, the same probably holds in most cases. Although the condition is not vertically transmitted because of its lethality, most cases examined have had heterozygous point mutations of COL1A1 or COL1A2 identified. Even though only heterozygous, these mutations appear to exert a dominant effect and badly disrupt collagen structure, because they prevent proper post-translational modification of the triple-helix molecules of which they are a part. (Several modifications to the procollagen molecule, including propeptide cleavage, lysine and proline hydroxylation, and cross-linking, are required for the collagen fibres to have the correct mechanical strength.)

This family would, therefore, be unusual if they do indeed have a recessive form of osteogenesis imperfecta.

What investigations were performed to confirm the diagnosis?

Collagen biosynthesis studies in fibroblasts cultured from the dead baby showed an aberrantly migrating α_1(I) chain. This was then followed up by analysis of the COL1A1 gene for mutations, allowing identification of a heterozygous mutation causing a glycine to arginine substitution at codon 667.

On analysis of DNA from both parents, the codon 667 mutation was not seen. This is not the expected finding for an autosomal recessive disease, but suggests rather that the amino acid substitution in their second child was the result of a new dominant mutation.

If both children had the same disorder, how can the recurrence of new dominant mutation be explained?

This situation strongly suggests the presence of gonadal mosaicism in one or other parent. To visualize the meaning of this term, consider where and when a new mutation might occur. Normally if a mutation is present in a parent it is passed on in the gametogenic cells (sperm or egg) during meiosis; the fertilized egg carrying the mutation will give rise to an individual who will have that mutation in every cell in his/her body (non-mosaic).

However, occasionally an embryo may start out its development genetically normal. If a mutation then occurs in one cell at an early stage of embryonic development, only the progeny of that cell will inherit the mutation whilst the other cells will not contain the mutation, resulting in a mature individual mosaic for normal and mutation-carrying cells. The mutation may be confined to only one or a few tissues. If one of these tissues in which the mutation occurs is a gametogenic precursor cell, the mutant cell line may be confined entirely to the gonad. This is called gonadal mosaicism. In such individuals the mutation is not present in other tissues and therefore the person is not clinically affected. In addition, as most DNA studies involve looking at DNA obtained from blood, the mutation will not be found as it is only present in the gonads. If the mutation is also found in some but not all somatic tissues (such as skin or blood), then the correct term is somatic and gonadal mosaicism.

Usually, gonadal mosaicism can only be inferred from the occurrence of events like those in our case. The recurrence risk for the disease in question can then only be guessed, since the proportion of abnormal gametes is unknown. If a mutation is found, as here, it may be possible to demonstrate that that mutation, though absent from blood DNA, is present in DNA extracted from sperm. This indeed proved to be the case. It was possible to estimate that between 15 and 20% of Damien's sperm carried the point mutation (suggesting that 30–40% of the spermatogenic cells were heterozygous for the mutation). This allowed the recurrence risk to be estimated at 15–20%, and prenatal diagnosis by chorionic villus sampling to be offered in future pregnancies.

QUESTIONS (ANSWERS ON PAGE 174)

1 Which of these statements applies to Fragile X syndrome?

a An abnormal FMR1 protein is produced in affected boys.

b Normal transmitting males can be detected cytogenetically.

c All daughters of a normal transmitting male are affected with Fragile X.

d Mosaicism is common in affected individuals.

e Point mutations can cause Fragile X syndrome.

2 The following are true of mitochondria and mitochondrial inheritance

a All mitochondrial proteins are encoded on the 16 kb mitochondrial genome.

b Almost all an individual's mitochondria are inherited from the mother.

c The genetic code is different in the mitochondrial and the nuclear genomes.

d Lactic acidosis is common in mitochondrial disorders.

e A mitochondrial DNA mutation is found in some diabetics.

3 Cryptic translocations

a Cryptic translocations can account for mental handicap in individuals who have had normal karyotypes.

b Fluorescent *in situ* hybridization can be used to detect cryptic translocations.

c DNA polymorphisms can be used to detect cryptic translocations.

d Male to male transmission does not occur in families with cryptic translocations.

e Only balanced carriers can transmit cryptic translocations.

4 Imprinted genes

a Imprinted genes are expressed from only one of the two alleles.

b Imprinted genes are randomly distributed in the genome.

c About a quarter of human genes are imprinted.

d Imprinted genes are only inherited from one parent.

e Imprinted genes show methylation differences between the two alleles.

5 Uniparental disomy

a always causes abnormality.

b is detected by routine cytogenetic analysis.

c can be demonstrated by use of DNA polymorphisms.

d may result in an abnormal methylation pattern demonstrable by Southern blotting.

e maternal and paternal UPD have been reported for all human chromosomes.

6 Gonadal mosaicism

a Can occur for X-linked mutations.

b Increases the recurrence risk for apparently new dominant mutations.

c Can be shown by analysis of DNA extracted from sperm.

d Is a common cause of infertility.

e Can occur for a chromosomal abnormality.

9

Cancer Genetics

LEARNING OBJECTIVES

After studying this chapter, the reader should understand:

- that tumorigenesis is a multi-step process
- the contribution of oncogenes, tumour suppressor genes and mutator genes to tumour development

- some specific familial cancer syndromes

INTRODUCTION

Cancer is a common condition affecting about 1 in 3 people sometime during their lifetime. The vast majority of cancers are sporadic developing from cells which have undergone somatic (or sporadic) alterations in their DNA structure, whilst the minority are due to an underlying germ-line (or inherited) mutation and are therefore truly 'genetic'. Since cancer is a common disorder, clustering of cases of cancer within families may be coincidental, genetic, or may reflect a shared environment or culture. Some cancers have strong environmental triggers, e.g. lung cancer and associated cigarette smoking, whilst other tumours such as bowel cancer, occurring in patients under the age of 30, are more likely to have a significant genetic basis. Even within families where there appears to be a strong genetic basis for the malignancies observed, it is still important to remember that some types of cancer commonly occur in individuals who are not carriers of the predisposing genetic mutation.

The majority of familial cancers whose underlying molecular pathology has been characterized involve the initial mutation of a tumour suppressor gene (**Box 9.1**), although many other types of genes become involved at later stages (**Box 9.2**). Loss of a functional copy of a tumour suppressor gene increases the individual's susceptibility to the development of a particular pattern of cancer, although the degree of susceptibility to individual cancers is dependent on the tumour supressor gene mutated, the specific mutation within that gene, as well as environmental interactions. For example a woman with an inherited mutation BRCA1 mutation (see Case 9.4) has an 85% breast cancer risk by age 70, whilst her risk of developing ovarian cancer may vary from 30% to 85% dependent on the BRCA1 mutation present.

BOX 9.1 TUMOUR SUPPRESSOR GENES

Genes normally involved in cell growth regulation, when abnormally activated or deactivated, have been associated with the development of cancer. Cancer is a form of independent aggressive evolution, involving the usual mechanisms of mutation and selection for cells with the mutation conferring a proliferative advantage.

Tumour suppressor genes

Originally known as anti-oncogenes, tumour suppressor genes appear to act as repressors of cell differentiation and proliferation. Inactivation of these genes allows abnormal cellular proliferation. Most are thought to conform to Knudson's 'two-hit' hypothesis, i.e. to act in a cellular recessive manner such that both copies of gene have to be inactivated for a cellular effect to occur, although exceptions have been described.

Knudson's 'two-hit' hypothesis

In 1971 Knudson published his now famous two-hit hypothesis to explain the pattern of tumorigenesis. The paradigm he used was retinoblastoma. The hypothesis states that specific inactivation events are needed in both copies of the RB1 gene before a tumour will develop. If there is a germ-line mutation in the RB1 gene, i.e. present in all cells, then this counts as the 'first hit'. Somatic mutational events may subsequently knock out the second copy of the gene in a particular retinoblast 'second hit', which then goes on to develop as a retinoblastoma. In individuals without a RB1 germ-line mutation, two somatic mutation events affecting RB1 are needed in the same retinoblast before a retinoblastoma develops (Fig. 9.1).

Although originally coined to explain retinoblastoma, the two-hit hypothesis has been shown to have a wider application as a model of tumour suppressor gene function in several inherited cancers and their sporadic counterparts.

Tumour suppressor genes involved in specific familial cancer syndromes

Gene	Syndrome
p53	Li Fraumeni
RB1	Retinoblastoma
BRCA1	Breast/ovarian cancer

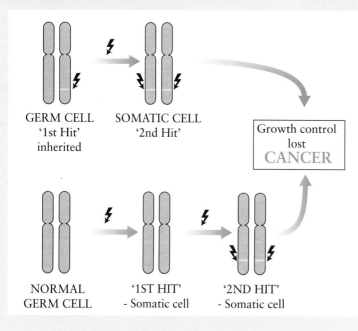

GERM CELL '1st Hit' inherited   SOMATIC CELL '2nd Hit'

Growth control lost
CANCER

NORMAL GERM CELL   '1ST HIT' - Somatic cell   '2ND HIT' - Somatic cell

Fig. 9.1 Knudson's two-hit hypothesis.

BOX 9.2 CANCER SUSCEPTIBILITY GENES

Cancer develops due to the involvement of multiple genes. These genes can be divided into:

(1) tumour suppressor genes (Box 9.1)

(2) proto-oncogenes

Oncogenes are derived from naturally occurring sequences in the genome known as proto-oncogenes. These genes are often growth factors, growth factor receptors, signal transducers or transcription regulators. Activation of these genes through mutation often increases abnormal unregulated proliferation of the cell. Their chief characteristic is the ability to transform cells. Oncogenes have a very important role in the development and subsequent behaviour of sporadic cancers through the mechanisms listed below.

◆ Impairment of normal regulatory elements (IGFRII in Wilms tumour)
◆ Amplification of production of oncoprotein product (N-myc amplification in neuroblastoma)
◆ Activation of a novel gene through chromosome translocation (**Box 9.3**)
◆ Production of an altered protein with transforming potential as a result of a gene mutation (mutations in k-RAS in many sporadic tumours)

Germ-line mutations leading to activation of an oncogene are extremely rare as many oncogenes are growth factors or growth factor receptors which have an important role in embryonic development. Thus mutations in these genes would be embryologically lethal. One exception is a rare familial cancer syndrome MEN Type 2 (multiple endocrine neoplasia type 2) which is associated with germ-line point mutations in the RET oncogene.

(3) Regulators of cell death

Bcl-2 functions by prolonging the lifespan of an individual cell by preventing apoptosis (programmed cell death). Pathological activation of Bcl-2 extends survival of a cell, thus providing opportunity for proto-oncogene activation or loss of tumour suppressor gene function.

FACTORS SUGGESTING A FAMILIAL BASIS TO THE CANCER

The following factors suggest a familial basis to the cancer:

● an earlier age of onset than would be expected for a particular tumour type
● several close relatives affected
● more than one primary tumour in the same individual (a primary tumour is one that does not arise as a result of spread from another tumour)
● a pattern of cancer fitting into a recognized cancer syndrome

Although in general inherited cancers form less than 1% of all cancers, they represent a high-risk group. The early detection of gene carriers opens up the opportunity of taking prophylactic measures to prevent the cancer developing, or detecting it early enough, through screening methods, for curative treatment to be possible. Some genetic cancers have an early premalignant form which can be treated to prevent future malignant conversion. For example, inheritance of a mutation in the adenomatous polyposis coli (APC) gene leads with near certainty to the development of premalignant colonic polyps. At this stage prophylactic surgery can be performed.

Case 9.1
Retinoblastoma

Family tree

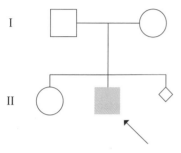

Presenting problem

Ben (II-2), aged 15 months, attended his health visitor because his mother was concerned that he was not doing as well as his sister had at the same age. The health visitor confirmed that his development appeared to be 'slow', and asked the GP's opinion. On examination the GP noticed that his right pupil 'looked white'. She arranged for him to be immediately reviewed by an ophthalmologist who diagnosed a right-sided retinoblastoma.

What is a retinoblastoma?

A retinoblastoma is an eye tumour which develops in embryonic retinal cells called retinoblasts (Fig. 9.3). The majority of these tumours develop in children under the age of 2 years although older children still have a small risk.

Retinoblastoma can be sporadic (60%) or genetic (40%). Genetic cases have a germ-line (heritable) mutation in a tumour suppressor gene RB1 on chromosome 13, and therefore have a risk of developing a second tumour in the other eye as well as tumours at other sites, especially osteosarcomas. All cases of bilateral retinoblastoma are due to germ-line mutations (see **Box 9.1**).

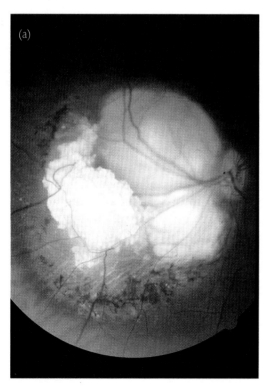

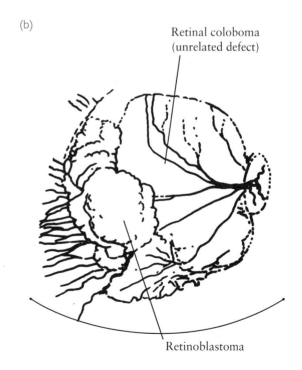

Fig. 9.3 Retinoblastoma. (Figure supplied by Ms Jan Johnson.)

Was Ben's retinoblastoma sporadic or genetic?

Ben had to have his right eye removed, although in some cases radiotherapy is sufficient treatment. There was no previous history of retinoblastoma in the family but, at his GP's request, blood was taken for chromosome analysis. The karyotype was reported as 46,XY,del(13)(q14), indicating that Ben has a germ-line deletion of the RB1 gene. Ben's parents' chromosomes were checked and found to be normal.

As Ben's mother is now pregnant, what are the risks of the new baby developing retinoblastoma?

About 3% of cases of retinoblastoma will have a cytogenetic deletion at chromosome 13q14, similar to Ben, which deletes the RB1 gene along with surrounding genes. Individuals with chromosome 13 deletions may in addition be mentally handicapped as part of a contiguous gene syndrome (Chapter 2, Box 2.3). The majority of these deletions arise *de novo* and the recurrence risk in siblings is therefore low if both parents have a normal karyotype. Although the risk is low, a recurrence of the deletion in a future pregnancy cannot be completely discounted as either parent could be a gonadal mosaic (Chapter 8). For this reason the newborn child would have his/her chromosomes checked soon after birth.

What follow-up should be arranged for Ben?

It is important that a child in whom a deletion has

BOX 9.3 RECIPROCAL TRANSLOCATIONS IN CANCER

Reciprocal translocations in cancer are thought to be somatic events that lead to a growth advantage to the carrier cell. These are likely to be important events in the multi-step process involved in the development of cancer. The best known example of a reciprocal translocation is the Philadelphia chromosome t(9;22) (q34;q11) (Fig. 9.2)

This results in fusion of genes on the maternal chromosome 22(BCR) and the paternal chromosome 9 (Abl) to create a single chimeric oncogenic protein product (BRC-Abl). Other examples of this phenomenon are:

◆ **acute promyelocytic leukaemia (APL)** – t(15;17)(q22;q11.2-q12) results in fusion of the MYL and RARA genes
◆ **synovial sarcoma** – t(X;18)(p11.2;q11.2) results in the fusion of the SSXT gene to either of 2 distinct genes, SSX1 or SSX2

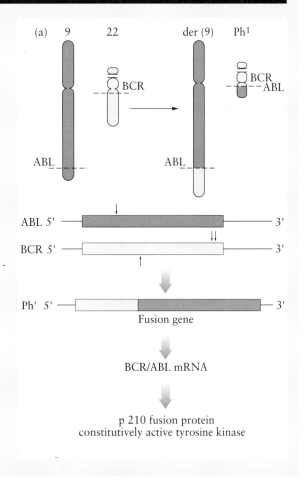

Fig. 9.2 The Philadelphia chromosome is a somatic, acquired translocation (t(9;22)(q34;q11) arising in chronic myeloid leukaemia. Translocation breakpoints lie within two specific genes *BCR* and *ABL*. The new *BCR-ABL* fusion gene produced by translocation encodes *ABL* tyrosine kinase.

been found, or who has a familial form of RB, has screening of the other eye as there is a significant risk of a second lesion developing. Early detection may allow sight-saving treatment to be performed. Ben will need to be screened by retinal examination 3-monthly to the age of 2, 6-monthly until the age of 5 and yearly until age 11. At first these examinations will require a general anaesthetic until he is able to understand and co-operate fully. Parents are also informed of the risk of associated osteosarcomas and therefore advised to take seriously any bony symptoms.

CASE 9.2
Familial adenomatous polyposis coli (APC)

Family tree

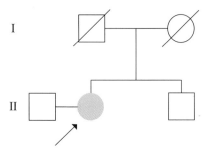

Presenting problem

Iris (II-2), aged 30, presented to her GP with rectal bleeding and abdominal pain. The GP referred her promptly to a surgeon who performed a colonoscopy which showed an ulcerating lesion on the wall of the ascending colon and the presence of multiple polyps (Fig. 9.4). A diagnosis of familial adenomatous polyposis coli was made and a colectomy (surgical removal of the colon) performed. Fortunately the pathology report did not show malignant change in the ulcerating lesion.

What is adenomatous polyposis coli?

APC is an autosomal dominant cancer syndrome characterized by the development of hundreds of polyps or overgrowths of the bowel wall, usually in the teenage years, which progress to multiple malignancies. It has an incidence of about

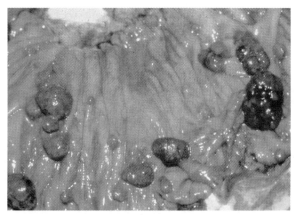

Fig. 9.4 Multiple polyps in familial adenomatous polyposis coli. (Figure supplied by Professor John Burn.)

1 in 8000 and is inherited as an almost completely penetrant autosomal dominant trait. About 70% of cases have a family history, whilst the remaining 30% are due to new mutations. Extra-colonic features, including benign tumours such as osteomas of the mandible and desmoids, are found in many gene carriers and these, may have fatal consequences due to local pressure effects. In many families, gene carriers have an unusual retinal lesion called a CHRPE (congenital hypertrophy of the retinal pigment epithelium) which causes no symptoms but can be used clinically to identify gene carriers (Fig. 9.5). Polyps can also develop in the upper part of the gastrointestinal tract where they are far harder to detect and treat than in the colon. Removal of the colon with an ileo-rectal

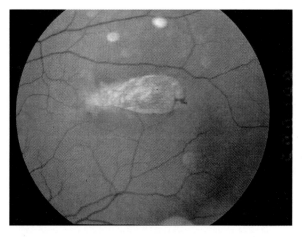

Fig. 9.5 Congenital hypertrophy of the retinal pigment epithelium. (Figure supplied by Professor John Burn.)

anastomosis is usually the first line of preventative treatment, followed by removal of the rectum at a later date. This will effectively remove the risk of a gene carrier developing a colonic malignancy. However, tumours can still develop in other parts of the digestive tract. Trials are underway in known APC gene carriers to see whether, by means of drug and diet modification, formation of colonic polyps and thus their need for surgery can be reduced (**Box 9.4**).

BOX 9.4 CAPP I AND TAMOXIFEN TRIALS

CAPP I trial

In 1993 the concerted action polyposis prevention study (CAPP) was established to conduct randomized controlled trials across Europe. The first study is evaluating the use of low dose aspirin and resistant starch in familial adenomatous polyposis coli gene carriers prior to their surgery. It is hoped that these treatments in combination will reduce polyp formation and thus requirement for surgery in gene carriers. There is a move to extend the study (CAPP II) to include the hereditory non-adenomatous polyposis coli gene carriers.

Tamoxifen trial

Tamoxifen is a drug which blocks the stimulatory effect of oestrogen on breast cancer cells. It has been used as a form of treament for breast cancer especially in postmenopausal women and has been shown to reduce the incidence of a new primary breast cancer in those with a previous breast cancer primary by about 40–50%. These findings have formed the basis of the trial using tamoxifen as prophylactic agent in women with a high familial risk of breast cancer.

Women at very high risk of developing breast cancer on family history alone are being recruited and randomized into receiving tamoxifen or placebo. It is hoped that as this group of women is followed up in the future the group receiving the tamoxifen will have a lower incidence of breast cancer.

What are the implications of Iris's diagnosis to the rest of her family?

As APC is an autosomal dominant condition, Iris's brother John (II-3) is also at risk of being affected. Examination of Iris's eyes showed that she had multiple CHRPE lesions in both retinae. John was offered ophthalmological screening which demonstrated that his retinae were clear of CHRPE lesions. He was therefore given a low risk of carrying the APC mutation responsible for the disease in his sister and this was later confirmed by DNA analysis when Iris's APC mutation was characterized.

What role does APC mutation detection play?

The APC gene is at chromosome 5q21 and the vast majority of the mutations found in APC families cause a loss of function of the gene. This strengthens the view that the APC gene is a tumour supressor gene (**Box 9.1**). In those families in which the disease is not associated with CHRPE, screening requires regular colonoscopies to detect the presence of polyps, an age-related phenomenon. APC gene mutation detection allows gene carriers to be identified in at-risk individuals prior to their developing polyps. Trials are currently underway to try and reduce the formation of polyps in known gene carriers (**Box 9.4**).

Specific mutation identification may also explain the variation in clinical phenotype. Individuals with a mutation in exon 15 have a severe phenotype with profuse polyps, whilst families with mutations affecting exon 9 onwards are associated with CHRPEs.

The gene for APC has been shown to play an important role in the development of sporadic bowel tumours as well as polyposis (**Box 9.5**).

BOX 9.5 BOWEL CANCER

Tumorigenesis is known to be a multi-step process. In 1990 Fearon and Vogelstein proposed a genetic model for colorectal tumorigenesis proceeding through a series of at least seven mutations. The accumulation of the mutational events is important rather than the order in which they occur. Mutator gene mutations (Case 9.3) increase the speed of mutation accumulation.

Pattern in the bowel	Genetic change
Normal epithelium	
↓	APC gene (gate keeper) allele loss
Hyperproliferation	
↓	DNA hypomethylation
Early adenoma	
↓	mutation in K-ras gene
Intermediate adenoma	
↓	DCC gene allele loss
Late adenoma	
↓	p53 gene allele loss
Carcinoma	
↓	other genetic change (mutations in tumour suppressor genes)
Metastasis	

CASE 9.3
Hereditary non-polyposis colorectal cancer (HNPCC)

Family tree

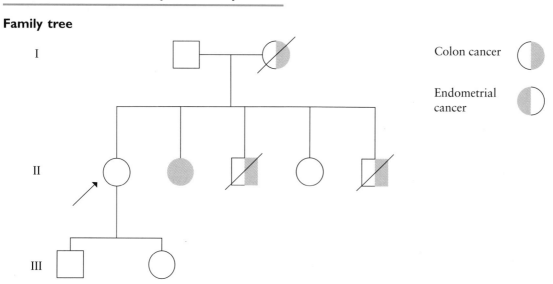

Colon cancer

Endometrial cancer

Presenting problem

Rosemary (II-1) attended the genetics clinic as she was worried about her family history of colon cancer.

Her mother (I-2) had died age 51 from cancer of the colon as had her two brothers Kyle (II-5) and Andrew (II-3), aged 22 and 30 respectively. Her sister Fiona had had a colectomy 3 years previously and had recently developed endometrial cancer. Rosemary is concerned regarding her own and her children's risk of developing colon cancer.

What is the most likely cause of colon cancer in Rosemary's family?

Hereditary non-polyposis colorectal cancer (HNPCC) is an autosomal dominant cancer syndrome. Families often have with a strong history of colon cancer, usually right-sided, with an early age at diagnosis. The colonic cancer is not preceded by the formation of thousands of polyps as seen in APC. In addition a subset of these families also have a predisposition to extra colonic cancers such as endometrial, ovarian and breast. Such families account for 3–6% of total annual colorectal cancers, thereby forming a larger group of familial colorectal cancers than APC.

What is the cause of HNPCC?

During cell division it is vital that DNA replication is accurate, preventing the accumulation of gene mutations, the hallmark of cancer. 'Proofreading' of replicating DNA and the correction of naturally occurring mutations are the functions of a set of genes called 'mutator genes' (**Box 9.6**). A mutation in one of these genes allows the accumulation of naturally occurring mutations in a cell and thereby increases the chance in that cell of a cancerous change. Tumours arising due to a mutator gene mutation are often RER (replication error) positive. This means the tumour shows a variation in microsatellite 'CA' repeat numbers (Chapter 4, **Box 4.2**) compared to the repeat number seen in peripheral blood DNA (Fig. 9.6). The 'CA' repeats have not been accurately copied during cell proliferation. The 'CA' repeat number was compared in DNA from a tissue section of Fiona's colon cancer and her blood DNA. This showed instability, strengthening the diagnosis of HNPCC in the family.

What is the significance of the diagnosis to Rosemary and her family?

Rosemary is at high risk of developing colon and endometrial cancer and therefore should be offered

---

BOX 9.6 MUTATOR GENES

Mismatch repair is a highly conserved celluar function carried out by gene products which recognize mismatched base pairs, excise them and then replace them with the correct bases. The genes involved in mismatch repair are called mutator genes and were originally described in bacteria. They include:

hMSH2	chromosome 2p22
hMLH1	chromosome 3p21.3
PMSL1	chromosome 2q31
PMSL2	chromosome 7q11

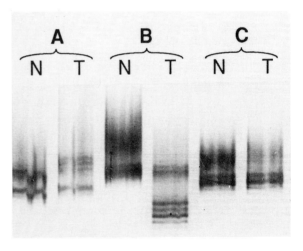

Fig. 9.6 Variation in microsatellite 'CA' repeat number in tumour (T) compared with the repeat number in peripheral blood DNA (N). Patients A and B are RER positive and C is negative. (Figure supplied by Mr Malcolm Dunlop.)

---

screening for this. Regular colonoscopy would be the favoured screening method for colon cancer and regular endometrial visualization and biopsy for endometrial cancer. As long as Rosemary does not develop cancer, the risk to her children is low.

Rosemary's younger sister should also be offered regular screening. If a mutation can be found in one of the mutator genes in Fiona's DNA, then Rosemary and her younger sister could be screened for the presence of this mutation and, if positive, future screening or surgery could be offered.

CASE 9.4
Breast and ovarian cancer

Family tree

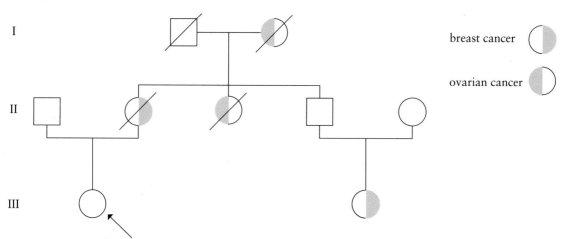

breast cancer

ovarian cancer

Presenting problem

Susan (III-1) is a 35-year-old nurse whose mother died of breast cancer at the age of 42. Her grandmother and aunt both died of ovarian cancer. In addition, Susan's cousin (III-2) has recently been diagnosed with breast cancer. Susan would like to know whether these cancers are connected, and has asked for genetic counselling.

Are these cancers likely to be connected and, if so, what is Susan's risk?

Breast cancer is a common disorder affecting ~1 in 12 women at some point in their lives and therefore it is not unusual to have more than one affected individual in a family. However, certain families have a particular predisposition to breast cancer which often occurs at an earlier age than in the rest of the population. In some of these families there is an increased incidence of ovarian cancer as well. So far two genes associated with breast cancer have been discovered, BRCA1 and BRCA2, on chromosomes 17q and chromosome 13q respectively. Mutations in BRCA1, a tumour suppressor gene, have been found in some families with both breast and ovarian cancer. Mutations in BRCA2 appear to occur in families with breast cancer but are less commonly associated with ovarian cancer. In a family such as Susan's, with four

or more affected individuals, the chance of there being an underlying genetic mutation in one of these genes is about 90%. The presence of two ovarian cancers in her family would make it more likely a BRCA1 mutation is present. If Susan is a carrier of a BRCA1 mutation her lifetime risk of developing breast cancer is 85% and the risk of developing ovarian cancer 30–80%, depending on the specific mutation present.

What options are available to Susan?

Breast and ovarian screening
Regular breast examination in association with 2-yearly mammography after the age of 35 may reduce the morbidity and mortality of breast cancer in familial cases by allowing early detection and intervention. Trials are underway to assess the efficacy of such screening. Ovarian screening by trans-vaginal ultrasound is as yet unproven but is being offered on a trial basis in some centres in association with annual serum CA125 measurement. Women at very high risk of breast cancer are also currently being enrolled in the tamoxifen trial (**Box 9.4**).

Direct gene testing
Although theoretically an option, mutation analysis in this family has logistic and technical prob-

lems. If blood can be obtained from Susan's cousin with breast cancer and DNA from a post-mortem specimen of tumour from her mother, grandmother or aunt, it may be possible to look for a BRCA1 or BRCA2 mutation in the family. If the mutation can be identified, then Susan could be offered presymptomatic testing (Chapter 5). If Susan tests negative for the mutation, then her lifetime risk of developing breast or ovarian cancer is not increased above that of the normal population, 8% and 1% respectively. However, the disease in Susan's family may not be due to a mutation in BRCA1 or 2, but to an as yet unidentified gene, in which case the absence of a mutation in either gene may be falsely reassuring. In large families the question may be solved using linkage (Chapter 4) to see whether in the particular family the cancer does link to BRCA1 or 2. Direct gene testing for BRCA1 and BRCA2 mutations is a very labour-intensive and costly technique as these genes are large and mutations can occur anywhere along

their length. At the present level of knowledge concerning the function of BRCA1 the interpretation of missense mutations (Chapter 3, Box 3.3) is difficult. There is no evidence for a common mutation in the non-Jewish population, akin to the ΔF508 mutation in cystic fibrosis.

Prophylactic surgery

Some women at high risk from a family history, as well as women who test positive for a BRCA1 or BRCA2 mutation, may opt for prophylactic mastectomy and/or prophylactic oophorectomy. Whilst this will lower the risk of developing cancer considerably, mastectomy is a major surgical procedure and may have many physical and psycho-social complications. In addition prophylactic oophorectomy in young women will also necessitate long-term hormone replacement therapy to prevent osteoporosis and does not totally negate the possibility of developing ovarian cancer.

CASE 9.5
Breast cancer

Family tree

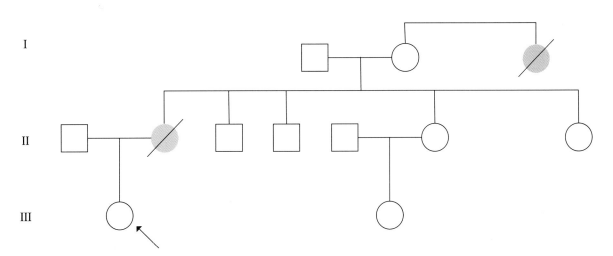

Presenting problem

Laura (III-1) is 27 years old. Her mother (II-2) died at the age of 60 of breast cancer which was diagnosed 3 years earlier. Laura has seen a recent TV documentary and is concerned because her

mother's aunt also died of breast cancer at the age of 81. In view of the family history Laura wishes to be screened.

Is Laura at increased risk?

Looking at Laura's family tree, a few key features are evident:

● Laura's mother was over 55 when her cancer was diagnosed.
● Her great aunt did not develop breast cancer until the age of 81. Breast cancer affects about 1 in 12 women over their lifetime.
● There are only two cases of breast cancer in this large family with several unaffected older women.

Laura's breast cancer risk is raised slightly because she has a first degree relative with breast cancer. Her great aunt's cancer does not affect this risk.

Should Laura be screened?

Breast and ovarian cancer are frequently the subject of articles in women's magazines and there is an expectation that screening for early disease and direct gene testing should be widely available. 'The New Genetics' is a popular topic for prime time TV science documentaries, leading to increased awareness of genetics but often to unrealistic expectations in the general public. Screening for early disease is an extremely controversial area, with medical experts openly disagreeing about the costs and benefits particularly to younger women. Screening for early breast cancer usually involves a mammogram causing exposure to a small amount of radiation. As the cumulative effect of such doses of radiation is not yet known, it has been argued that there is no justification for mammography in young women (under 40 years of age). Additionally there is no good evidence that mammography in this age group is effective in detecting early tumours. Other screening modalities such as ultrasound are generally not thought sufficiently sensitive for widespread use.

Laura is in a low-risk group on family history and of an age where mammography is not of proven benefit as a screening modality. The standard procedure is therefore that she should be counselled on the basis of her risk and taught breast self-examination. It is important that she does not feel that her fears have been trivialized or that she is being denied screening on economic grounds.

A national programme does exist for breast screening in women over the age of 50, as this has been proven to be of clinical value.

CASE 9.6
von Hippel Lindau syndrome

Family tree

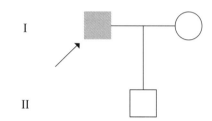

Presenting problem

James (I-1) presented to his GP at the age of 26 with blackouts and severe headaches which wakened him at night. He was referred to a neurologist who organized a CT scan. The scan showed a space-occupying lesion in his cerebellum (Fig. 9.7). At surgery the tumour was found to be a haemangioma. As 50% of cerebellar haemangiomas are associated with von Hippel Lindau syndrome (vHL), an ophthalmological assessment was carried out which showed a small haemangioma on the right retina. A diagnosis of vHL was made.

What is von Hippel Lindau syndrome?

vHL is an autosomal dominant inherited cancer syndrome due to mutations in a tumour suppressor gene on chromosome 3p. A wide variety of tumours have been described in affected individuals, the commonest being retinal angioma and cerebellar, spinal and brain stem haemangioblastomas. Somatic mutations in the same gene have also been implicated in sporadic renal tumours.

What follow-up should be offered to James?

Carriers of mutations in the vHL gene are offered a series of screening tests aimed at early detection

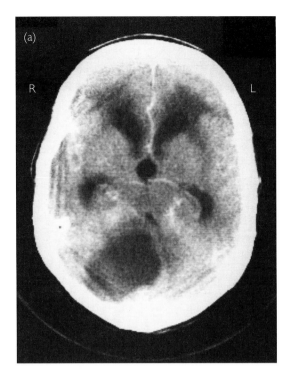

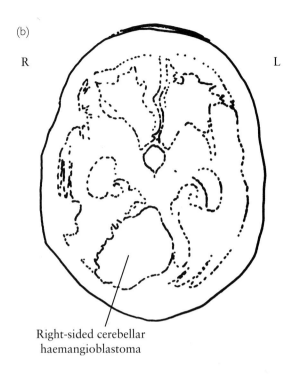

Right-sided cerebellar
haemangioblastoma

Fig. 9.7 Haemangioma associated with von Hippel Lindau syndrome.

of tumours. Regular ophthalmological examination will detect retinal haemangiomas which are then treated to prevent loss of vision. Abdominal ultrasound scanning should be performed yearly so that renal tumours (clear cell carcinomas) can be picked up early. vHL is also associated with tumours of the adrenal gland called phaeochromocytomas and these can be screened for by a urine test. In addition, 3-yearly cranial MRI scans should be performed to detect any further tumours which may develop.

What is the clinical implication of the diagnosis for John's son Frank?

As vHL is an autosomal dominant condition, Frank (II-1) has a 1 in 2 risk of having inherited the condition, and therefore should also be offered a similar screening regimen from the age of 16. If a mutation is identified in James's vHL gene then presymptomatic testing will be available to Frank.

CASE 9.7
Ataxia telangiectasia

Family tree

I

II

Presenting problem

Jenny (II-1), an 8-year-old girl, was referred to the paediatrician because of frequent falls and a 'nervous tic'. Her mother had died from breast cancer and Jenny was currently living with foster parents. Close examination of Jenny's eyes showed telangiectases (small tortuous blood vessels) on the sclerae (white of the eye). This finding, in conjunction with the clinical symptoms, suggested the diagnosis of ataxia telangiectasia (AT), and for this reason the paediatrician took blood for karyotyping and alphafetoprotein (AFP) analysis, normally only present at low levels in the non-pregnant woman. The chromosome analysis showed multiple chromosomal breaks and translocations, and the AFP was elevated. A diagnosis of AT was confirmed in Jenny.

What does the future hold for Jenny?

AT is an autosomal recessive chromosome breakage syndrome (**Box 9.7**).

Jenny may have been ataxic (unsteady on her feet) for some time before anyone became aware of it. The ataxia is progressive and affected children are frequently wheelchair-users by their teenage years. Children with AT have an increased susceptibility to malignancies, in particular leukaemias and lymphomas.

Is the history of breast cancer in Jenny's mother significant?

It has been hypothesized but not yet established that the 1 in 150 women who are heterozygous carriers for a mutation in the AT gene are at three times population risk of developing breast cancer. This is not proven as it is difficult to identify AT carriers.

FURTHER READING

Hodgson SV, Maher ER (1993) *A Practical Guide to Human Cancer Genetics*. Cambridge University Press, Cambridge.

BOX 9.7 CHROMOSOMAL BREAKAGE SYNDROMES

Chromosome breakage syndromes such as ataxia telangiectasia, Fanconi anaemia and Bloom syndrome are rare autosomal recessive errors of DNA repair associated with tendency to malignancy, particularly leukaemias. These conditions can usually be diagnosed on the basis of the specific pattern of chromosome breakage seen when cells are cultured and exposed to environmental stress in the form of UV light, irradiation or certain chemicals.

Ataxia telangiectasia (AT)

AT is characterized by a progressive ataxia, scleral telangiectases and immunodeficiency and is caused by mutations in the ATM gene on chromosome 11q23. Affected individuals have a high serum AFP (Fig. 9.8).

Fanconi anaemia (FA)

FA is characterized by the development of severe anaemia, a low white cell and low platelet count as a result of bone marrow failure. Children with the condition may have a variety of malformations and patchy pigmentary changes in the skin. The condition shows locus heterogeneity with a major locus at chromosome 16q24 (Fig. 9.9).

Bloom syndrome

Bloom syndrome is characterized by growth retardation, both pre- and post-natally, a sun-sensitive rash and pigmentary skin abnormalities. The gene for Bloom syndrome has been mapped to chromosome 15q25.

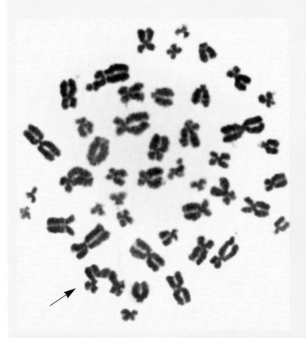

Fig. 9.8 Unbanded metaphase spread from patients with AT showing multiple chromosome breaks. Arrow shows triradius. (Figure supplied by Mrs Elizabeth Grace.)

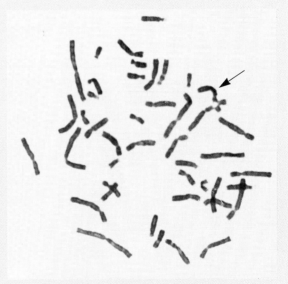

Fig. 9.9 Unbanded metaphase spread from patients with Fanconi anaemia. Arrow shows quadriradius. (Figure supplied by Mrs Elizabeth Grace.)

QUESTIONS (ANSWERS ON PAGE 175)

1 Familial cancer syndromes

a make up a small proportion of all cancers.

b can be dominant or recessive.

c can be associated with p53 mutations.

d tend to present at a younger age than sporadic cancer.

e are usually associated with chromosome translocations.

2 Breast cancer

a occurs at a younger age in BRCA1 carriers than in sporadic cases.

b is a common feature of von Hippel Lindau syndrome.

c is usually associated with germ-line BRCA1 mutations.

d can be caused by germ-line BRCA2 mutations.

e screening is only available to women at increased genetic risk.

3 Mutations in

a mutator genes may lead to bowel cancer.

b the Ras oncogene family are usually inherited.

c BRCA1 may cause ovarian cancer.

d somatic cells accumulate with age.

e p53 may cause lung cancer in smokers.

4 Direct gene testing

a is possible for most individuals with a family history of breast cancer.

b is possible for most individuals with a family history of familial adenomatous polyposis coli.

c can be carried out routinely in most hospital laboratories.

d should only be performed with the patient's consent.

e is usually performed on DNA.

5 Chromosome breakage syndromes

a may be associated with an increased risk of breast cancer.

b are associated with DNA repair defects.

c may cause congenital malformations.

d are usually dominantly inherited.

e are the commonest cause of cancer in childhood.

6 Knudson's two-hit hypothesis

a may provide an explanation for BRCA1 action.

b describes the mechanism of action of oncogenes.

c refers to loss of function in two alleles.

d is important in colon cancer.

e refers to the inactivation of oncogenes.

10

Birth Defects and Syndrome Identification

LEARNING OBJECTIVES

After studying this chapter, the reader should understand:

- the classification of patterns of birth defects
- the range of normal physical growth
- the importance of embryology in understanding birth defects
- how to investigate the dysmorphic child

INTRODUCTION

Dysmorphology is the clinical study of abnormal physical development with the aim of understanding the causes of human birth defects. This speciality covers a bewildering array of diagnoses (currently >2000) which reflects the complexity of human development. This involves a remarkable series of events culminating in the structural and functional attainment of the adult state from a single fertilized egg cell. As with all physiological processes there is considerable normal variation within and between populations in the size and shape of a normal individual. A knowledge of prenatal and postnatal physical variation is, therefore, vital in dysmorphology and some examples of normal ranges in important growth parameters are given in **Box 10.1**.

Dysmorphology assessment is usually requested in a child with one or more congenital anomalies. Between 2 and 4% of live births have some form of birth defect, most of which can be categorized as:

- **malformations** – intrinsic defects in the pattern of development e.g. structural cardiac abnormalities (Case 10.1), conjoined twins (Case 10.2), neural tube defects (Case 10.3)
- **deformations** – abnormal development of a structure caused by extrinsic forces, e.g. abnormal head shape due to intrauterine 'squashing' (Case 10.4)
- **disruptions** – destruction of a normally formed tissue, e.g. amniotic bands causing limb amputations.

A specific diagnosis can only be made in around a third of cases. Of these:

- ~ 10% are due to chromosomal anomalies.
- ~ 22% single-gene defects, e.g. Waardenburg's syndrome (Case 10.5), Smith–Lemli–Opitz syndrome (Case 10.6).
- ~ 5% teratogenic agents (chemical agents with a malign influence on development, e.g. cocaine, ethanol, warfarin, anticonvulsants (Case 10.7).

In the remaining two-thirds of cases the cause is

BOX 10.1 CLINICALLY IMPORTANT GROWTH PARAMETERS

In most growth charts a line corresponding to the mean and 2.57 standard deviations above and below the mean are plotted against age. Measurements falling outside these limits (3rd and 97th centile lines) are generally considered to be significantly abnormal (Fig. 10.1).

◆ **linear growth** – change in body length over time (growth velocity) is a useful measurement. Many genetic diseases, particularly chromosomal anomalies, are associated with short stature and poor growth velocity which begins in intrauterine life. Genetic disorders of the skeleton may result in disproportionate short stature where the growth velocity of particular body segments is affected more than others. An example of this would be the shortening of the limbs compared with the trunk and head in achondroplasia.

◆ **weight** – some genetic diseases, such as Prader–Willi syndrome (Chapter 8) and Bardet–Biedl syndrome (autosomal recessive disorder with polydactyly, mental handicap) may cause obesity.

◆ **head circumference** – is important as it is an indirect measurement of brain growth. Microcephaly is a common feature of many genetic diseases and can reflect poor brain growth (e.g. de Lange syndrome) or premature fusion of the skull sutures (craniosynostosis, usually with unusual head shape). An abnormally large head circumference may reflect hydrocephalus (increased intracranial fluid pressure, e.g. X-linked hydrocephalus) or increase brain growth (e.g. Sotos syndrome).

◆ **facial growth** – normal facial growth is simple to recognize but difficult to describe. The most

(a)

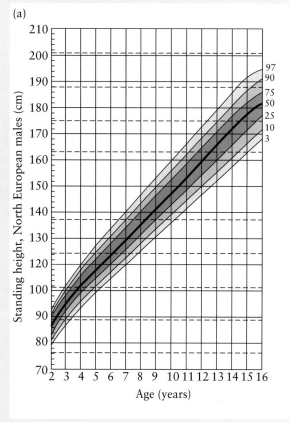

(b)

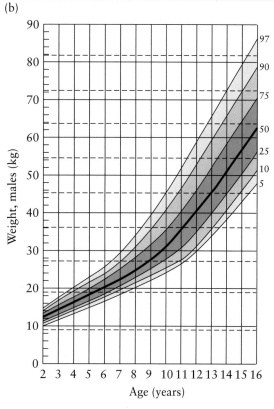

BOX 10.1 CLINICALLY IMPORTANT GROWTH PARAMETERS (Cont.)

(c)

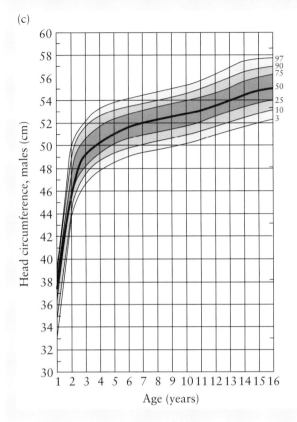

(d)

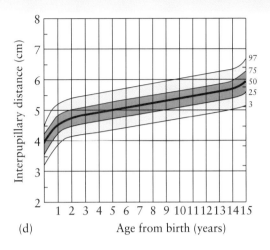

Fig. 10.1 Growth charts (male). (a) linear growth (standing height); (b) weight; (c) head circumference; (d) intrapupillary distance. From Tanner and Whitehouse (a); Hamill *et al.* (b); Nellhaus (c); and Feingold and Bossert (d).

commonly used facial measurements relate to eye shape and the distance between ocular landmarks.

◆ Blepharophimosis is a reduction in the length of the palpebral fissure and is a feature in ~100 different syndromes and is often seen in fetal alcohol syndrome.

◆ Hypertelorism is an increased distance between the orbits and is a feature of almost 400 different syndromes including the Aarskog syndrome (hypertelorism, digital abnormalities and short stature).

◆ Hypotelorism is a reduced distance between the orbits and is a feature of >40 different syndromes including holoprosencephaly (incomplete separation of the frontal lobes of the brain).

◆ Telecanthus is an increased distance between the inner canthi with either normal or abnormal interorbital distances and is a feature in ~90 different syndromes such as Waardenburg's syndrome (see Case 10.5).

unknown. In such cases an attempt should be made to estimate where and when the developmental insult occurred during embryogenesis. The pattern of organs affected may be particularly useful in this regard as these may be derived from a common tissue of origin, e.g. teeth, hair, skin and nail abnormalities in ectodermal dysplasias. **Box 10.2** describes a useful system for categorization of patterns in congenital anomalies.

BOX 10.2 PATTERNS OF BIRTH DEFECTS

◆ **single-site defects** – these involve one organ system only and make up the majority of children with birth defects, e.g. cleft lip, microphthalmia, anencephaly (Case 10.3)

◆ **associations** – this is the non-random association of groups of congenital anomalies but in a relatively inconsistent manner, e.g. CHARGE association (coloboma, *h*eart defects, *a*tresia of the choana (occlusion of the nasal passages), *r*etardation of growth, *g*enital anomalies, *e*ar anomalies), schisis association (NTD, orofacial clefts, omphalocoele and diaphragmatic hernia) and VACTERL (see Case 10.1)

◆ **sequences** – where a single site defect results

in other apparently unrelated anomalies due to a developmental cascade this is termed a sequence, e.g. Potter's sequence (see Case 10.4)

◆ **developmental field complex** – this is a situation where abnormalities in adjacent structures of disparate embryological origins are seen together, e.g. hemifacial microsomia

◆ **syndromes** – if a combination of birth defects is consistent in unrelated individuals then this may be called a syndrome. There are currently >2000 syndromes described. Many of these do show some phenotypic variation both in individuals throughout life (developing phenotype) and between different individuals.

CASE 10.1
VACTERL association

Family tree

Presenting problem

A paediatric surgeon has referred a 5-week-old male child, Fraser (Fig. 10.2), who has had a successful surgical repair of a tracheo-oesophageal fistula. Several other malformations had been noticed in this baby including a ventricular septal defect and bilateral renal dysplasia. A chest X-ray showed upper thoracic vertebral abnormalities. Externally Fraser had a missing left thumb and hypoplasia of the left radius. His face and cranial examination were normal and his chromosomes revealed normal 46,XY. A genetic referral was made as Fraser's mother wants to know if a future child would be similarly affected.

What is the diagnosis?

Finding the correct diagnosis in a child with multiple congenital abnormalities requires careful clinical evaluation and a systematic method used to construct a list of differential diagnoses (**Box 10.3**). The pivotal features in Fraser's case are the missing thumb and tracheo-oesophageal fistula and by searching computer dysmorphology databases a list of differential diagnosis such as:

● VACTERL association
● Nager acrofacial dysostosis (unusual face, malformed ears and radial aplasia)
● Fanconi anaemia

is suggested. In view of the normal facial features and presence of vertebral abnormalities the likely diagnosis in this baby is the VACTERL association. This is an acronym for *V*ertebral anomalies, *A*nal atresia, *C*ardiac defects, *T*racheoo*E*sophageal fistula, *R*enal anomalies and *L*imb defects. The cause of VACTERL is not known. Approximately 15% of infants with tracheo-oesophageal fistulae have features of VACTERL association. It is a relatively well-known condition and in reality could be diagnosed by most experienced paediatricians and clinical geneticists without use of computer databases. However, if the above case had hydrocephalus in addition to the features described rarer associations and syn-

(a)

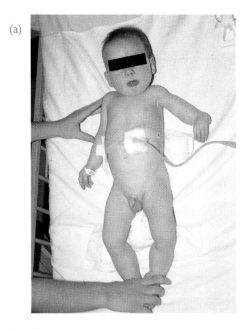

(b)

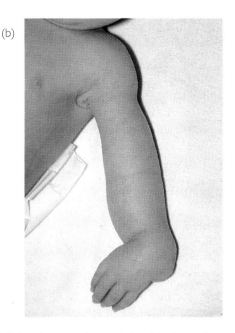

Fig. 10.2 (a) Successful repair of a tracheo-oesophageal fistula. (b) Missing thumb and hypoplasia of the left radius.

BOX 10.3 MAKING DIAGNOSES IN DYSMORPHOLOGY

The following systematic approach is useful:

- **family tree** – evidence of malformations or health problems in other members of the family may considerably help in making a diagnosis (see Cases 10.5 and 10.6).
- **pregnancy history** – evidence of drug exposure (Case 10.7) or infectious illnesses (e.g. rubella, toxoplasmosis, cytomegalovirus, varicella) may explain a pattern of birth defects.
- **physical examination** – detecting both major and minor birth defects may allow better use of pivotal features. These are clinical clues which are unusual enough in isolation or combination to allow the diagnostic search (either computer- or brain-based) to be narrowed enabling correct diagnosis.
- **investigations** – these must obviously be tailored to the particular case but the following are frequently used in dysmorphology:
  - chromosome analysis (Chapter 2)
  - skeletal survey – many conditions show defects in bony development
  - brain imaging – the ability to detect anatomical abnormalities in brain structure during life has been a major advance in dysmorphology

- dermatoglyphic analysis – detects abnormalities in the formation of the ridges present in the skin particularly over the palms and soles of the feet.
- **differential diagnosis** – >2000 different dysmorphic diagnoses have now been described, all of which are rare and some have been reported only once. For these reasons it is very difficult for most clinicians to retain all the necessary information to diagnose all cases. Syndrome and association identification, like many branches of medicine, is basically an exercise in pattern recognition of pivotal features. For this reason several groups have developed computerized databases to *aid* in the identification of specific dysmorphic diagnoses. These programs all work by matching the features of the case under investigation against those of known syndromes stored in a database. These programs have proven to be very useful but in practice are aids for and not replacements of experienced clinicians. Details of some of these programs are given in the Further reading section.
- **conclusion** – in at least half the cases a diagnosis cannot be reached and the clinician must not be afraid to admit this. The wrong diagnosis will help no-one.

dromes should be considered. By studying such a computer database it can be seen that a rare disorder called Fanconi anaemia can occasionally present as VACTERL syndrome with hydrocephaly. Fanconi anaemia is a serious autosomal recessive disorder of DNA repair characterized by pancytopaenia, skin pigmentation and a predisposition to malignancy (Chapter 9, Box 9.7). This condition was excluded in Fraser by demonstrating that he did not have the characteristic increase in chromosomal breaks in response to exposure of the cultured cells to mitomycin C *in vitro*.

What is the reproductive risk and prognosis in a future pregnancy?

The risk of VACTERL occurring again in a future pregnancy is relatively low (<2%). Unfortunately, ~25% of children with VACTERL die during infancy mostly as a consequence of their heart anomalies. It was important to have ruled out Fanconi anaemia in Fraser as this would have a 1 in 4 recurrence risk as an autosomal recessive condition.

CASE 10.2
Conjoined twins

Family tree

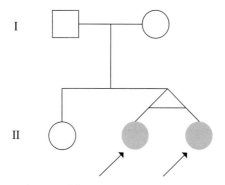

Presenting problem

Louise and Charlotte were born by emergency caesarian section at 36 weeks' gestation. They were the children of a travelling family who had not booked for antenatal care. At birth they were joined by their thorax and abdomen (Fig. 10.3). Investigations showed that they shared a single and

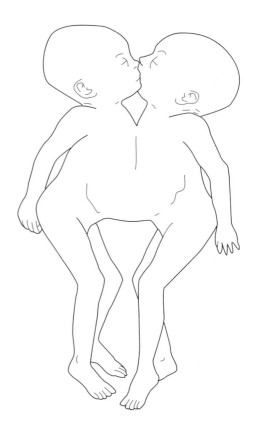

Fig. 10.3 Conjoined twins. These twin girls are joined by their thorax and abdomen.

grossly abnormal heart. After extensive discussion involving the parents it was decided that any attempt to separate the twins surgically would be unsuccessful and should not be attempted. In view of the very poor outlook the parents expressed a wish to take the twins home where they died 24 hours later.

How did this anomaly arise?

Conjoined twins are rare and result from an extremely early abnormality in human development as a complication of monozygous twinning. Monozygous (identical) twinning occurs at a rate of ~4 per 1000 births (**Box 10.4**) and is due to the complete cleavage of the inner cell mass of the blastocyst in the preimplantation period (**Box 10.5**) whilst dizygous (DZ) or fraternal twinning resulting from fertilization of two different eggs and occurs in ~1 in 120 pregnancies). Rarely in

BOX 10.4 TWINNING

Dizygous (DZ) twins share ~50% of their genetic material whereas monozygous (MZ) twins are genetically identical. The study of twins has proven to be a very useful way to assess whether a disease has a genetic component to its aetiology. The basis of these studies is that most twins share a common environment at least in intrauterine and early postnatal life. Therefore, if you can identify a group of MZ and DZ twins where one twin has developed condition x, if more MZ co-twins also develop x (twin concordance) than DZ co-twins it suggests that there is a significant and measurable genetic contribution to the aetiology of that disorder. The genetic contribution to a disease. can then be quantified using a calculation of heritability. The higher the MZ concordance, the greater the genetic component of the disease. Some examples of twin studies are given in Table 10.1.

Table 10.1 Twin studies

Disorder	MZ % concordance	DZ % concordance
Peptic ulcer	53	36
Myocardial infarction (males)	39	26
Myocardial infarction (females)	44	14
Non-insulin dependent diabetes mellitis	70	15

monozygous twinning splitting of the single embryo can be incomplete which results in conjoined twins. The anatomical site of joining depends on the site of the cleavage in relationship to the established polarity of the embryo. These twins are also called Siamese twins after Eng and Chang, the 'united twins of Siam'.

BOX 10.5 PREIMPLANTATION PERIOD OF HUMAN DEVELOPMENT (GESTATIONAL DAY 1–7)

Fertilization usually occurs in the ampullary region of the fallopian tubes. Subsequent mitotic cell divisions create first a ball of cells (the morula, day 2–3) and then a hollow sphere (the blastocyst, day 4) with a small mound of cells on the inner aspect of this sphere (the inner cell mass) from which the embryo will develop. Up until this point there has been almost no overall growth accompanying these cell divisions (Fig. 10.4). On ~day 5–6 there is attachment of the embryo to the endometrium and by day 7 the blastocyst has implanted in the uterine wall, gaining a new source of nourishment which allows for a rapid and sustained period of growth. Monozygous twinning is the only human 'disorder' which dates specifically to the preimplantation stage of development.

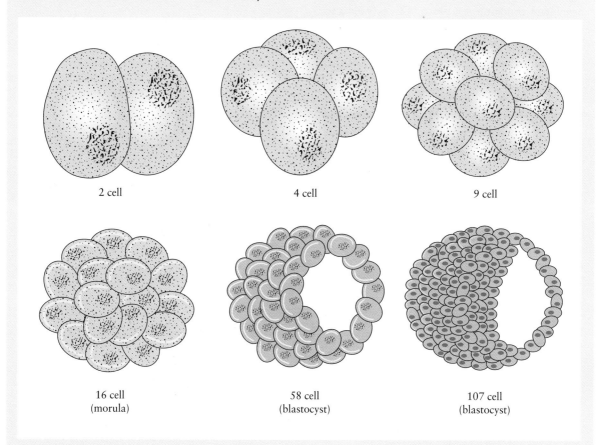

2 cell   4 cell   9 cell

16 cell (morula)   58 cell (blastocyst)   107 cell (blastocyst)

Fig. 10.4 Preimplantation development of the human embryo.

CASE 10.3
Anencephaly

Family tree

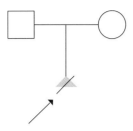

Presenting problem

Angela is 16 years old and presented to hospital at 22 weeks' gestation after a concealed pregnancy. A detailed ultrasound scan showed a male fetus with a severe abnormality of the skull vault and brain (Fig. 10.5; Chapter 6, Box 6.1). The scan was indicative of anencephaly and in view of this Angela decided to terminate the pregnancy 3 days later.

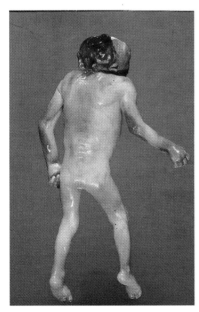

Fig. 10.5 Anencephaly.

What causes anencephaly?

The neural tube is an important structure that forms in the embryonic period of development (**Box 10.6** and Chapter 6, Fig. 6.2). Failure of the neural tube to fuse completely results in two main types of malformation collectively called neural tube defects (NTD). Anencephaly is caused by failure of the anterior neuropore (the gap at the cranial end of the neural tube) to close on day 24. Failure of the caudal neuropore to close on day 26 results in spina bifida. These malformations show several very interesting features:

● significant familial clustering – the risk of recurrence of a NTD in a future pregnancy (without treatment) is 2–4%
● geographical variation – there is a birth incidence of NTD of ~1 in 300 in Ireland and <1 in 1000 in the USA
● remarkable changes in incidence over time – NTD incidence has fallen in Scotland from 1 in 300 in 1975 to 1 in 700 in 1995
● maternal folate supplementation in the periconceptual period reduces the likelihood of NTD recurrence by 75%
● prenatal diagnosis of NTDs can be successfully performed using biochemical screening (for raised maternal serum AFP) and detailed ultrasound scanning (see Chapter 6, Box 6.1)

What is the explanation for the vitamin response?

It is now thought that differences in folate metabolism underlie the development of NTD. In particular, presence of a variant heat-labile form of the enzyme methylenetetrahydrofolate reductase appears to confer a susceptibility to NTD. It is likely that this metabolic abnormality can be partly overcome by either dietary or pharmacological supplementation with folate.

BOX 10.6 EMBRYONIC PERIOD (GESTATIONAL DAY 8–~56)

After implantation the cytotrophobast invades the endometrium and will ultimately form the placenta. By day 10 the embryo has developed into a plate-like structure made up of two layers of cells; the ectoderm and the primitive endoderm. On the surface of the ectoderm a linear indentation called the primitive streak forms and, in a process called gastrulation, ectodermal cells migrate toward and then down through the primitive streak. The first cells to pass through the primitive streak replace the primitive endoderm with embryonic endoderm. The next wave of migrating cells forms a layer between the ectoderm and the endoderm called the mesoderm. These three primitive embryonic tissues (also called the germ layers) will each contribute the majority of cells to a different set of body structures (Table 10.2). At this stage the embryo has already established polarity, i.e. which end will be the head end. Several other important processes occur in very early development before the onset of true organogenesis.

◆ **notochord formation** – a central rod of cells forms in the mesoderm along the length of the embryo at ~day 16. The notochord has a central role in inducing the development of the nervous system by sending chemical signals which cause differentiation of cells in the overlying ectoderm.

◆ **the neural tube** – one of the first regions of specialization within the embryo is the thickened region on the dorsal ectodermal surface called the neural plate. Elevation of the lateral edges of the neural plate form the neural groove and approximately halfway along the groove the edges fuse in the midline. Between days 22–26

fusion spreads in both cranial and caudal directions giving rise to the neural tube. Elements of the neural tube later form the brain and spinal cord. Failure to complete closure at the cranial and caudal end results in anencephaly and spina bifida respectively (Case 10.3). Collectively these defects are known as neural tube defects.

◆ **neural crest cells** – a very important group of cells which behaves as a fourth germ layer. These cells form on the lip of the neural plate and migrate throughout the body to give rise to pigmentary and nerve cells and many of the structures that determine the shape of the face (Table 10.2).

◆ **somite development** – between days 20 and 28 approximately 30 segmental blocks of tissue form in the midline mesoderm along the back of the embryo called somites. Cells from this process give rise to the vertebral bodies and muscle and dermis of that particular body segment.

Table 10.2 The embryonic origins of adult tissues

Germ layer	Adult tissue
Ectoderm	Brain, spinal cord, retina, skin, nails, hair, lens and cornea of eye, oronasal epithelia, tooth enamel, inner ear
Neural crest	Adrenal medulla, schwann cells, melanocytes, facial bones and muscles, parasympathetic ganglia
Mesoderm	Skeletal muscle, heart and blood vessels, limbs, axial skeleton, urogenital system, adrenal cortex
Endoderm	Gastrointestinal system, bladder, respiratory epithelium

CASE 10.4
Potter's sequence

Family tree

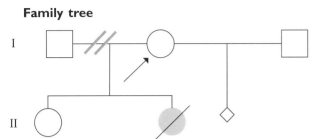

Presenting problem

Caroline (I-2) is now 10 weeks' pregnant. Her previous child, Terri (II-2), by a different partner, died at the age of 1 hour. A post-mortem report showed that this baby had bilateral absence of the kidneys (renal agenesis) with flattened nose, low-set ears and hypertelorism. There was severe underdevelopment of the lungs which was the cause of death. Amnion nodosa was present (a nodular appearance to the amniotic membranes). Chromosome analysis in Terri showed 46,XX normal karyotype. Caroline wished to know if this problem would occur again in this pregnancy.

What was the diagnosis in Terri?

The clinical features in Terri are diagnostic of Potter's sequence. This phenotype is secondary to severe, prolonged oligohydramnios (lack of amniotic fluid) and is often seen in association with bilateral renal agenesis. Unilateral renal agenesis is seen in 1 in 1000 births and is usually asymptomatic. Bilateral renal agenesis affects ~1 in 3000 births and is incompatible with life. The embryonic basis of this defect appears to be in the failure of induction of mesoderm by the ureteric bud during organogenesis (**Box 10.7**); the cause of this failure is not known. Approximately 10% of first degree relatives of children with bilateral renal agenesis have an asymptomatic renal malformation suggesting that there may be a significant genetic basis to the aetiology. Throughout most of pregnancy the amniotic fluid is formed by fetal urinary output, therefore, many severe renal malformations will result in oligohydramnios. In affected pregnancies there is squashing of the fetus causing the features mentioned above. Thus Potter's sequence is a malformation (renal agenesis) causing secondary deformations (flattened nose, low-set ears and lung hypoplasia).

BOX 10.7 ORGANOGENESIS

Organogenesis is a general term for the formation of specialized stuctures within the embryo. Some of the major events in organogenesis of the face, limbs and kidney which relate to common malformations are discussed briefly below.

Facial structures

The overall shape of the face is determined by the growth and fusion of various facial processes (Fig. 10.6):

◆ **frontonasal mass** – on day 28 an area of thickened ectoderm forms on the frontonasal mass called the nasal placode which subdivides it into:
  ◆ a nasomedial process which forms the nose and the central part of the upper lip
  ◆ paired nasolateral processes which will form the lateral nasal structures and fuse with the maxillary process along the nasolacrimal groove

◆ **bilateral maxillary processes** – form from one end of the 1st branchial arch, grows medially and fuses with the nasomedial process on day 40 to produce the upper lip. Failure of this process occurs in ~1 in 1000 births and produces cleft lip (Fig. 10.7).

◆ **bilateral mandibular processes** – forms from the other end of the 1st brachial and fuse in the midline on day 40 to produce the mandible.

Limbs

All four limbs arise in a similar way (Fig. 10.8):

BOX 10.7 ORGANOGENESIS (Cont.)

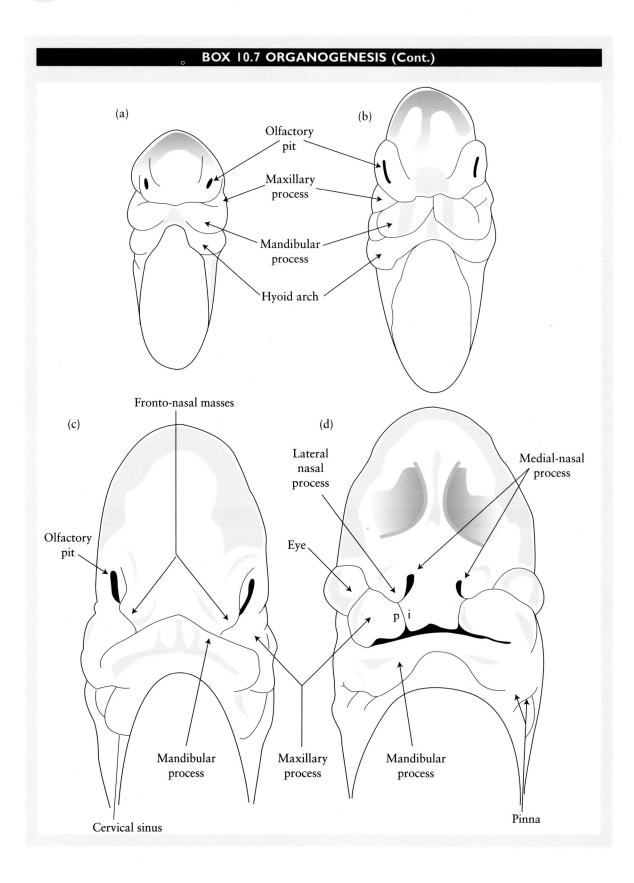

BOX 10.7 ORGANOGENESIS (Cont.)

Fig. 10.6 *(Right)* Development of the central face from the frontal process and the paired maxillary and mandibular processes. (a) Human embryo at early stage 12 with the primitive mouth bordered rostrally by the frontal process, laterally by the maxillary processes and caudally by the mandibular processes. (b) Late in stage 12 the mandibular processes enlarge until the growth centres are adjacent in the midline. (c) In stage 13 the mandibular processes fuse and the fronto-nasal mass becomes more distinct. (d) In stage 16–17 the medial nasal ridge and the intermaxillary processes (i) can be distinguished as separate growth centres. The intermaxillary centres will fuse with the premaxillary centres (p) late in stage 17.

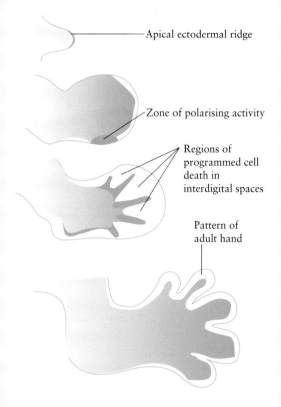

Apical ectodermal ridge

Zone of polarising activity

Regions of programmed cell death in interdigital spaces

Pattern of adult hand

Fig. 10.8 Limb development.

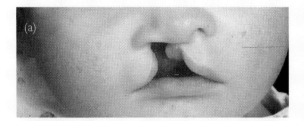
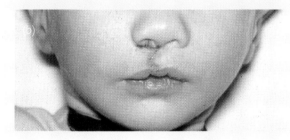

Fig. 10.7 Cleft lip.

◆ **apical ectodermal ridge** – at ~26 day for the upper limbs and day 28 for the lower limbs a thickening in the surface ectoderm of the lateral body wall appears called the apical ectodermal ridge. This induces and directs growth in the underlying mesenchymal tissue to produce the limb bud.

◆ **ZPA** – on day 33 flattened regions at the end of the limb buds appear called the hand and foot plates with development of a specialized area on one side of the plate apical ectodermal ridge called the zone of polarizing activity (ZPA). The ZPA induces the natural asymmetry in human limbs by signalling the thumb to develop on one side of the limb bud.

◆ **cell death** – regions of cell death appear on the hand and foot plate creating the interdigital spaces. Failure of this programmed cell death will

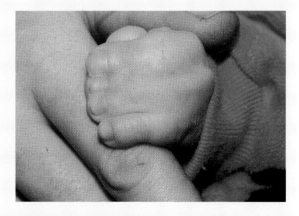

Fig. 10.9 Syndactyly.

BOX 10.7 ORGANOGENESIS (Cont.)

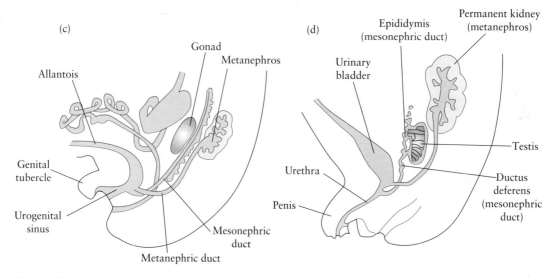

Fig. 10.10 Stages in the formation of the metanephros. (a) At 6 weeks; (b) at 7 weeks; (c) at 8 weeks; (d) at 3 months, male.

result in syndactyly (finger webbing or fusion) (Fig. 10.9).

Kidney

The human kidney develops in three main stages (Fig. 10.10):

◆ **nephrotomes** – these are transient structures consisting of cords of epithelial cells of mesodermal origin which appear on day 22. They connect with the primary nephric duct which grows towards the cloaca (the caudal opening of the primitive gut). The nephrotomes begin to degenerate by day 30.

◆ **mesonephros** – the primary nephric duct induces the formation of mesonephric tubules and the mesonephric duct which connects with the cloaca by day 28. Mesonephros is structurally similar to the glomerular and collecting systems

---

BOX 10.7 ORGANOGENESIS (Cont.)

found in fish. The mesonephros begins to degenerate by day 56 although in males the mesonephric duct is 'salvaged' as the epididymis and ductus deferens.

◆ **metanephros** – the ureteric bud develops

as an outgrowth of the distal mesonephric duct and induces the surrounding mesoderm to form the structure of the definitive kidney, the metanephros. Failure of this induction results in renal agenesis (see Case 10.4).

What is the recurrence risk in another pregnancy?

The risk of recurrence is 3–4% after bilateral renal agenesis. Prenatal diagnosis is possible using detailed ultrasound scanning (see Chapter 6, Box 6.1).

CASE 10.5
Waardenburg syndrome

Family tree

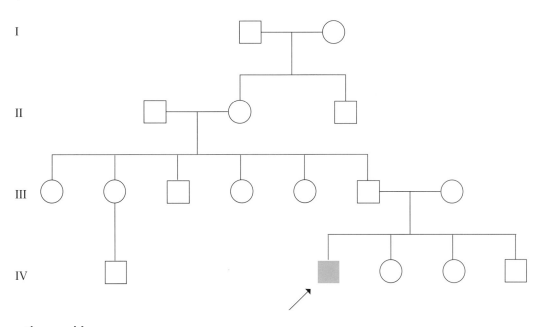

Presenting problem

Lawrence (IV-2) has been referred from the community paediatrician aged 4 years with a severe bilateral *sensorineural hearing loss*. At the clinic he was also noted to have other minor abnormalities, *heterochromasia* (different coloured eyes) and *telecanthus* (lateral deviation of the canthi) but an otherwise normal examination. Although no other members of the family had any medical problems or hearing problems when assessed, individuals III-2 and III-6 had *poliosis* (white forelock), IV-1 died with a diagnosis of Hirschprung's disease and II-2 and I-1 had early graying of their hair. On audiometric testing III-6 had unilateral sensorineural hearing loss.

Background

The diagnosis in this family is Waardenburg syndrome. The pivotal features which led to the diagnosis were the deafness, abnormal pigmentation (poilosis and heterochromasia) and the intestinal neuronal migration arrest (Hirschprung's disease). There are two types of Waardenburg syndrome, Type I is due to mutations in the *PAX3* gene on 2q37 and Type II due to mutations in the *MITF* gene on 3p12. Both these loci are thought to interfere with the migration or function of neural crest-derived cells which produce melanocytes, intestinal nerve supply and contribute cells to the inner ear.

What are the reproductive risks?

Waardenburg syndrome is an autosomal dominant condition with a 50% genetic risk to the offspring of an affected individual. However, this condition shows highly variable penetrance and there is currently no way to predict severity of the disease using DNA testing.

CASE 10.6
Smith–Lemli–Opitz syndrome

Family tree

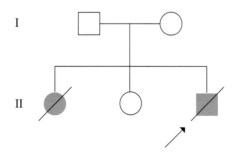

Presenting problem

A 1-day-old baby (II-3) was referred with the following collection of malformations: cleft palate, ambiguous genitalia, polydactyly (extra digit or digits), 2–3 syndactyly in both feet and unilateral renal agenesis (Fig. 10.10). This child had a sister

(II-1) who died 4 years before with a similar pattern of problems. Chromosome analysis in II-2 revealed a normal 46,XY karyotype and plasma cholesterol was 1.1 μmol/l (normal 3–6 μmol/l). II-2 died at the age of 10 days and post-mortem examination revealed an abnormal accumulation of 7-dehydrocholesterol in all tissues examined. Post mortem tissue from II-1 was retrieved and showed an identical abnormality.

Mechanism of disease

The pivotal features in this case are the polydactyly and ambiguous genitalia. The diagnosis in this case is Smith–Lemli–Opitz syndrome type II (SLO II). This is an autosomal recessive deficiency of an enzyme called 7-dehydrocholesterol reductase, an enzyme which catalyses the final step in the conversion of cholesterol from lanosterol. It is not, as yet, known whether it is the presence of 7DHC or the lack of cholesterol which is pathological and the embryological basis of the condition is not clear. SLO II is almost invariably fatal in the first month of life. A less severe form of this disorder, Smith–Lemli–Opitz type I (SLO I), can present later in childhood with developmental delay, ptosis and hypospadias in males. SLO type I also shows the accumulation of 7DHC which can be detected in plasma samples. This case also demonstrated the importance of storing post-mortem tissue from children like II-1 with unexplained malformations.

What is the reproductive risk?

The recurrence risk for future pregnancies is 1 in 4 or 25%. Prenatal diagnosis is available by analysis of the sterol content of chorionic villus biopsy or amniotic fluid.

Is there a treatment?

In the milder variant of this condition, SLO I, treatment of children with a high-cholesterol diet has been reportedly beneficial with regards to improving the developmental profile. It is extremely unlikely that such treatment will be of use or indeed desirable in view of the other severe abnormalities seen in SLO II.

CASE 10.7
Fetal valproate

Family tree

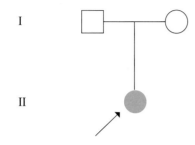

Presenting problem

Brigit has significant learning difficulties and unusual facial features characterized by a long philtrum with shallow orbits. She was otherwise in good health. The only relevant family history is that Brigit's mother, Gillian (I-1), has ideopathic epilepsy and has been taking sodium valproate for seizure prophylaxis for the last 6 years. Brigit's chromosomes showed a 46,XX normal karyotype.

Mechanism of disease

This is a situation where both the family history and the history of drug exposure during pregnancy has proven very useful in making the diagnosis. It is likely that the problems that Brigit has are related to exposure to sodium valproate during pregnancy. This was supported by comparison of Brigit's facial features with those of other children with valproate embryopathy. It is often the case in dysmorphology that subtle changes in facial morphology can give a syndrome a particular 'look'. Down syndrome is such a disorder. It is often described as the affected children looking more like each other than they do their own siblings. Details of this and other teratogenic effects are given in **Box 10.8**. The exact cause of the embryonic defect induced by valproate is not known.

What is the reproductive risk?

There is a significant risk of neural tube defects in women taking valproate during pregnancy. The risk of other features is not known although it may

---

BOX 10.8 TERATOGENIC AGENTS IN HUMANS

Up to 5% of congenital anomalies are thought to be due to exposure to environmental mutagens e.g.:

Viral:

◆ Rubella – microcephaly, cataracts
◆ Varicella – limb aplasia, body wall defect, eye abnormalities

Chemical:

◆ Alcohol – growth retardation, short palpebral fissures, smooth philtrum, microcephaly
◆ Cocaine – brain defects, puffy eyelids and growth retardation
◆ Lithium – cardiac defects
◆ Methotrexate – now rare, was seen when abortion was induced by folate antagonists, prominent eyes, limb shortening
◆ Retinoic acid – craniofacial, limb and brain defects
◆ Thalidomide – severe limb defects
◆ Valproate – neural tube defects, polydactyly and unusual face
◆ Warfarin – hypoplastic nose, chondrodysplasia punctata

---

be as high as 25%. However, folate supplementation is thought to reduce the risk of NTD. There are no clear guidelines on anticonvulsant use in pregnancy as phenytoin and carbemezepine also have teratogenic effects.

REFERENCES

Feingold M, Bossert WH (1974) Normal values for selected physical parameters: an aid to syndrome delineation. *Birth Defects: Original Article Series*, **X(13)**: 1–15.

Hamill PV, Drizd TA, Johnson CL, Reed RB, Roche AF, Moore WM. (1979) Physical growth: National Center for Health Statistics percentile.

American Journal of Clinical Nutrition, **32**: 607–29.

Nellhaus G (1968) Head circumference from birth to eighteen years. Practical composite international and interracial graphs. *Pediatrics*, **41**: 106–14.

Tanner JM, Whitehouse RH (1973) Height and weight charts from birth to 5 years allowing for length of gestation. *Archives of Disease in Childhood*, **48**: 786–89.

FURTHER READING

Aase JM (1990) *Diagnostic Dysmorphology*. Plenum Publishing, New York.

Buyse ML (1990) *Birth Defects Encyclopaedia*. Blackwell, Oxford.

Carlson BM (1994) *Human Embryology and Developmental Biology*. Mosby, St Louis.

Gorlin RJ, Cohen MM, Levin LS (1990) *Syndromes of the Head and Neck*. OUP, Oxford.

Jones KL (1988) *Smith's Recognisable Patterns of Human Malformations*. WB Saunders, Philadelphia.

Winter RM, Barraitser M (1995) *The London Dysmorphology Database Version 3*. OUP, Oxford.

WWW sites of interest

- **OMIM** – online Mendelian inheritance in man: a comprehensive catalogue of genetic diseases (http://www.hgmp.mrc.ac.uk/omim/searchomim.html)
- **DDB** – dysmorphology discussion board: a specialist site for case presentations and discussion (http://genetics.ich.bpmf.ac.uk/DDB/ddb.html)
- **Mouse–human dysmorphology database** – an attempt to link the many well-characterized mouse mutants to human model diseases (http://www.hgmp.mrc.ac.uk/DHMHD/dysmorph.html)

QUESTIONS (ANSWERS ON PAGE 175)

1 Syndrome diagnoses
a describe relatively consistent patterns of abnormalities.
b number >2000 different conditions.
c are often eponymous.
d usually involve local abnormalities in adjacent tissues of different embryological origins.
e imply a specific pathophysiology in most cases.

2 The neural tube
a forms by fusion of the lips of the neural groove.
b defects are usually caused by folic acid excess.
c fuses in a progressive cranial to caudal direction.
d defects involving the anterior neuropore cause anencephaly.
e defects may be caused by sodium valproate.

3 Human teratogenic effects
a from sodium valproate may cause digital anomalies.
b from ethanol are seen in 1 in 50 000 births.
c are not known for any vitamins.
d warfarin may result in chondrodysplasia punctata.
e usually act in the first 2 weeks after fertilization.

4 Monozygous twins
a are often conjoined
b share the same percentage of genes as double-first cousins.
c can be studied to calculate the genetic contribution to common disorders.
d with an adult-onset genetic disease will always develop symptoms at exactly the same age.
e have an increased risk of birth defects.

5 Limb development
a is apparent by 18 days of gestation.
b may be interrupted by teratogens.
c involves programmed cell death.
d begins in the lower limbs first.

e requires a ZPA on the thumb side of the hand plate.

6 The developing kidney
a is primarily derived from ectoderm.
b contributes to the male genital tract.
c is deformed in Potter's sequence.
d is morphologically complete by 38 days of gestation.
e is an uncommon site for human malformations.

7 Birth defects
a occur in 3 in 1000 live births.
b are almost all due to known chromosomal and single-gene defects.
c in most children involve only one organ system.
d are common in chromosomal abnormalities.
e always involve malformations.

8 Preimplantation period of development
a is accompanied by remarkable growth of the embryo.
b involves formation of the inner cell mass.
c is when most malformations occur.
d lasts ~2 weeks.
e can be partly accomplished *in vitro*.

9 Computer programs to aid dysmorphic diagnoses
a allow searches of combinations of birth defects.
b are best used when searching with pivotal features.
c are able to match facial photographs.
d are particularly useful in very rare disorders.
e should be used only as a last resort.

10 The diagnostic features of
a a sequence are restricted to a single anatomical site.
b a dysplasia are likely to be progressive.
c a syndrome are always birth defects.
d hemifacial microsomia are due to defects tissues derived from one germ layer.
e many syndromes show considerable overlap.

Appendix I

Accessing Information on Genetic Disorders

INTRODUCTION

Clinical genetics is a rapidly expanding speciality and the progress in our understanding of the molecular basis of inherited disorders is likely to continue apace. One reason for this optimism is that an international scientific collaboration called the Human Genome Project aims to determine the sequence of the entire human genome in the next 10 years. Even if this goal is not realized, there is no doubt that the volume of information available to clinicians will dramatically increase and it is unlikely that traditional paper-based reference texts will suffice. Therefore, an increasing reliance on electronic multimedia data sources should be expected. Up-to-date information is vital to optimize diagnostic and therapeutic approach to an individual patient. On-line databases (**Box A.1**) and current periodicals should be considered a more appropriate source of specific information on diagnosis and treatment for these rare disorders. The reader should try comparing the information available on-line with that given in Appendix II to appreciate the importance of vigilance and the dangers of complacency in clinical practice.

BOX A.1 ON-LINE DATABASES

◆ OMIM – on-line Mendelian inheritance in man (http://www.hgmp.mrc.ac.uk/omim/searchomim.html); a catalog of all Mendelian disorders in humans founded by Dr Victor McKusick, Johns Hopkins Hospital.

◆ HGMP – human genome mapping project (http://www.hgmp.mrc.ac.uk/); a collection of programs and databases of human genomic information.

◆ LDB – location database (http://cedar.genetics.soton.ac.uk/public_html/); an integrated database of chromosomal order of polymorphic sequences and genes.

◆ ENTREZ – (http://www3.ncbi.nlm.nih.gov/Entrez/); a search program that links the public databases of human genomic information with the scientific citations about each entry.

◆ GDB – genome database (http://www.hgmp.mrc.ac.uk/gdb/gdbtop.html); a catalog of all mapped human DNA sequences.

◆ EBI – European bioinformatics institute (http://www.ebi.ac.uk/); access to nucleotide and protein databases.

◆ Human Genome Project Information – general information on the quest to sequence the genome (http://www.ornl.gov/TechResources/Human_Genome/home.html).

◆ Link Pages – (http://www.hgmp.mrc.ac.uk/Public/human-gen-db.html).

Appendix II

Important Genetic Diseases

INTRODUCTION

There are currently >4000 different Mendelian genetic disorders described, all of which are individually rare. Collectively they affect about 1% of the population. This appendix provides some basic information on the disorders more frequently seen in clinical genetic practice. As stated in Appendix I, up-to-date information on all these disorders may be found in on-line public databases such as OMIM
(http://www.hgmp.mrc.ac.uk/omim/searchomim.html).

AUTOSOMAL DOMINANT DISORDERS

Connective tissue disorders and skeletal dysplasias

Marfan syndrome
- *incidence* – ~1 in 10 000.
- *genetic pathology* – most cases caused by mutations in the fibrillin gene on chromosome 15q, although at least one family is caused by mutations in an unknown gene on chromosome 3.
- *clinical features* – affects three main systems; the heart (mitral valve prolapse, dissecting aortic

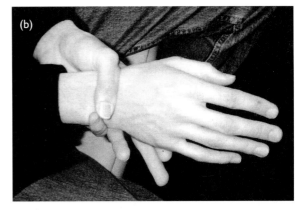

Fig. A.1 (a) Arachnodactyly in Marfan syndrome. Long thin tapering fingers. (b) Wrist sign in Marfan syndrome. The ability to wrap thumb and 5th finger around the wrist so that they overlap indicates arachnodactyl.

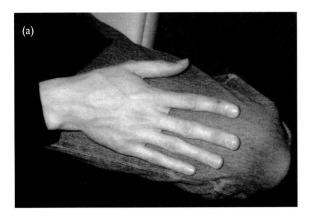

aneurysm), the skeleton (tall stature, scoliosis, arachnodactyly (Fig. A.1)) and the eyes (lens dislocation). Regular screening of the heart by echocardiography or MRI scan is recommended and prophylaxis using β blockers may prevent aortic root dilatation.

Ehlers–Danlos syndrome
- *incidence* – ~1 in 10 000
- *genetic pathology* – in most cases unknown but genetic heterogeneity suspected. Type IV is due to mutations in *COL3A1* gene (2q).
- *clinical features* – highly variable disorders with skin fragility and elasticity (Fig. A.2) and joint hypermobility (Fig. A.3) which has been divided into >10 different types on the basis of severity and primarily affected system. Type IV is particularly important as it has a high risk of vascular rupture leading to early death.

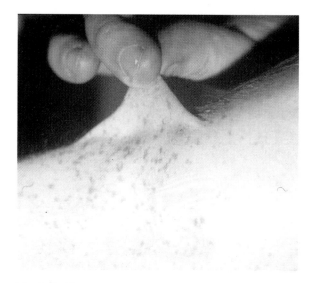

Fig. A.2 Skin elasticity in Ehlers–Danlos syndrome.

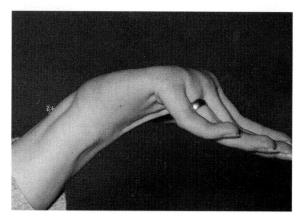

Fig. A.3 Joint hyperextensibility found in Ehlers–Danlos syndrome.

Osteogenesis imperfecta
- *incidence* – ~1 in 10 000.
- *genetic pathology* – caused by mutations in the COL1A1 gene on chromosome 17q or COL1A2 on chromosome 7q. Most cases autosomal dominant some appear to be recessive.
- *clinical features* – highly variable phenotype involving multiple fractures and bone deformity. Type I have blue discoloration of the sclerae and hearing loss. Type II is a perinatally lethal form of the disorder with poor boney mineralization (Chapter 8, Fig. 8.9). Type III is the severe progressively deforming type. Type IV have relatively mild disorder with short stature and dental abnormalities. Many of the more severe phenotypes are new mutations.

Achondroplasia
- *incidence* – ~1 in 10 000.
- *genetic pathology* – caused by mutations in the FGFR3 gene on chromosome 4p, most cases are new mutations.
- *clinical features* – generalized skeletal dysplasia causing marked limb shortening, macrocephaly and digital abnormality (trident hand, Chapter 3, Fig. 3.8). Homozygocity for this mutation leads to a neonatally lethal short-limb disorder.

Genodermatoses

Neurofibromatosis type I
- *incidence* – 1 in 3000.
- *genetic pathology* – caused by mutations in the neurofibromin gene on chromosome 17q. Eighty per cent of cases are new mutations.
- *clinical features* – characterized by light brown patches (café-au-lait patches) and lumps (dermal neurofibromas) on the skin (Fig. A.4), macrocephaly, scoliosis and learning difficulties in ~30% of children. Serious medical complications can arise from compression from internal neurofibromas.

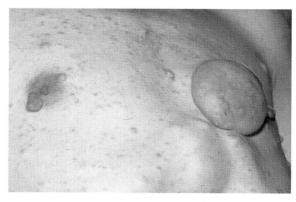

Fig. A.4 Café-au-lait patches and neurofibroma in a patient with NFI.

Neurofibromatosis type II
- *incidence* – 1 in 50 000.
- *genetic pathology* – caused by mutations in the merlin gene on chromosome 22q.
- *clinical features* – bilateral acoustic neuromas and early cataract formation are the hallmarks of this condition. Early detection of acoustic neuromas using MRI scanning may improve surgical preservation of hearing.

Tuberous sclerosis
- *incidence* – 1 in 15 000
- *genetic pathology* – caused by mutations in the tuberin gene on chromosome 16p and an unknown gene on 9q.
- *clinical features* – highly variable disorder characterized by cortical tubers in the brain, depigmented macules (ash leaf spots, Fig. A.5) and raised lesions (angiofibromas and shagreen patches) on the skin. Renal (angiomyolipoma) and lung lesions (lymphangioleiomyoma) are also seen. Severe mental handicap and epilepsy are common complications of this disorder.

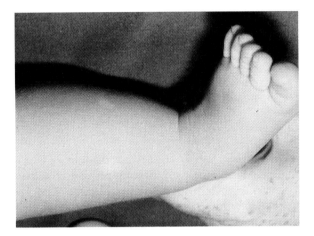

Fig. A.5 Ash leaf spots characterization of tuberous sclerosis.

Inherited Cancer Syndromes (see also Chapter 9)

Multiple Endocrine Neoplasia type 1
- *incidence* – rare.
- *genetic pathology* – caused by mutations in an unknown gene on chromosome 11q.
- *clinical features* – characterized by familial clustering of hyperparathyroidism, hyperinsulinism and prolactinomas.

Multiple endocrine neoplasia type 2
- *incidence* – rare.
- *genetic pathology* – caused by mutations in the Ret oncogene on chromosome 10q.
- *clinical features* – characterized by familial clustering of pheochromocytoma, medullary thyroid carcinoma and parathyroid adenoma.

Von Hippel Lindau
- *incidence* – 1 in 50 000.
- *genetic pathology* – caused by mutations in the tumour suppresser gene VHL on chromosome 3p.
- *clinical features* – characterized by cerebellar and spinal cord haemangioblastomas (Chapter 9, Fig. 9.7), retinal angiomas, phaeochromocytomas and renal cell carcinomas. Regular screening of at-risk individuals is recommended.

Neurodegenerative disorders

Adult onset cerebellar ataxia
- *incidence* – 1 in 20 000.
- *genetic pathology* – as expected there is marked locus heterogeneity. Spinocerebellar ataxia (SCA) type 1 is caused by mutations in the ataxin gene on chromosome 6p. SCA type 2, 3, 4 and 5 map to chromosomes 12q, 14q, 16q and 11 respectively. There are likely to be several other loci.
- *clinical features* – adult-onset progressive cerebellar ataxia often associated with ophthalmoplegia and dementia.

Huntington's disease
See Chapter 5, Case 5.5.

Neuromuscular Abnormalities

Myotonic dystrophy
- *incidence* – 1 in 9000.
- *genetic pathology* – caused by a (CAG) trinucleotide expansion mutation in the DM kinase gene on chromosome 19p.
- *clinical features* – progressive muscle weakness with myotonia (on inability to relax muscle tone normally), cataracts, cardiac conduction defects and hypogonadism.

Facio-scapulo-humeral dystrophy
- *incidence* – 1 in 50 000.
- *genetic pathology* – caused by an unusual mutation affecting an unknown gene on chromosome 4q.
- *clinical features* – progressive limb girdle and facial weakness particularly affecting the shoulder muscles.

Hereditary motor and sensory neuropathy type I
- *incidence* – 1 in 3000.
- *genetic pathology* – caused by a duplication of chromosome 17p including the PMP22 gene.
- *clinical features* – characterized by slow nerve conduction velocities, pes cavus, clawing of the toes and often a relatively benign clinical course.

Haematological disorders

Acute intermittent porphyria
See Chapter 5, Case 5.2.

Hereditary spherocytosis
- *incidence* – 1 in 5000.
- *genetic pathology* – caused by mutations in the ankrin-1 gene on chromosome 8p.
- *clinical features* – in this condition red cells appear spherical rather than biconcave discs. This results in a haemolytic anaemia which may require splenectomy.

AUTOSOMAL RECESSIVE DISORDERS

Dysmorphic syndromes

Smith–Lemli–Opitz syndrome
- *incidence* – 1 in 30 000.
- *genetic pathology* – deficiency of 7-dehydrocholes-terol reductase (7DHCR), an enzyme involved in the synthesis of cholesterol. The gene encoding this enzyme has not been identified.
- *clinical features* – in the neonatally lethal form of this disorder (type II) the common features are micro-cephaly, congenital heart defect, renal dysplasia, cleft palate and polydactyly. There is a less severe form (type I) which may present with mental handicap, ptosis and genitourinary malformations.

Zellweger syndrome
- *incidence* – 1 in 50 000.
- *genetic pathology* – caused by mutations in about nine different loci resulting in defects in the structure and function of peroxisomes.
- *clinical features* – raised plasma levels of very-long-chain fatty acids associated with severe developmen-tal delay, hypotonia, renal and hepatic malfunction.

Eye diseases

Retinitis pigmentosa
- *incidence* – ~1 in 4000.
- *genetic pathology* – remarkable genetic heterogene-ity; where no other abnormalities are found, 50% of cases are autosomal recessive, 15% autosomal dom-inant, 5% X-linked and the remainder of unknown inheritance pattern. More than 10 different genes known to be involved.
- *clinical features* – characterized by night blindness, constrictions of visual fields and 'spotty' pigmenta-tion of the retina. RP can be part of many different genetic syndromes.

Immunodeficiencies

Adenosine deaminase deficiency
- *incidence* – 1 in 100 000.
- *genetic pathology* – caused by mutations in the ADA gene chromosome 20q.
- *clinical features* – deficiency of this enzyme results in a severe immunodeficiency causing recurrent infec-tions. Treatment is available using bone marrow transplantation, enzyme replacement or gene therapy.

Ion Transport Defects

Cystic fibrosis
See Chapter 4, Case 4.1.

Inborn Error of Metabolism

Phenylketonuria
See Chapter 5, Case 5.1.

Classical galactosaemia
- *incidence* – 1 in 55 000.
- *genetic pathology* – caused by mutations in the GALT gene on chromosome 9. Seventy per cent of disease alleles carry the same mutation (Q188R).
- *clinical features* – often presents in the first week with vomiting, hepatomegaly, jaundice and oedema. Cataracts and mental handicap can be later clinical features. The diagnosis is made by measuring red cell galactose-1-phosphate uridyltransferase activity. Treatment uses a galactose-free diet.

Medium chain acyl CoA dehydrogenase deficiency
- *incidence* – 1 in 10 000.
- *genetic pathology* – caused by mutations in the MCAD gene on chromosome 1p. Approximately 90% of disease alleles carry the same mutation (K329E).
- *clinical features* – presents in the first few years of life with low blood glucose in response to infection or starvation with an inability to produce ketones. The diagnosis is often made on urinary excretion pat-terns of fatty acid conjugates.

Neurodegenerative disorders

Ceroid lipofuscinosis
- *incidence* – 1 in 150 000.
- *genetic pathology* – shows locus heterogeneity. Mutations have been identified in the PPT gene on chromosome 1p and the CLN3 gene on chromosome 16p.

● *clinical features* – onset in infancy or middle childhood with rapid deterioration in vision and dementia leading to early death.

Neuromuscular disorders

Spinal muscular atrophy
● *incidence* – 1 in 10 000.
● *genetic pathology* – caused by complex mutations in the SMN gene on chromosome 5q.
● *clinical features* – the most severe form (type I or Werdnig–Hoffman) presents with progressive weakness and hypotonia in the first few months of life caused by anterior horn cell degeneration and leading to death in infancy.

Metal transport disorders

Haemochromatosis
● *incidence* – 1 in 400.
● *genetic pathology* – caused by mutations in the HLA-H gene on chromosome 6p.
● *clinical features* – clinical features are the result of excess iron deposition in tissues, particularly the liver (causing cirrhosis) and pancreas (causing diabetes). Many cases are asymptomatic and serious complications can be avoided by regular venesection (blood donations).

X-LINKED RECESSIVE DISORDERS

Haematological

Haemophilia A
Haemophilia B
See Chapter 7, Case 7.1.

Immunodeficiencies

Severe combined immune deficiency
● *incidence* – rare.
● *genetic pathology* – caused by mutations in IL2RG gene (Xq). Obligate female carriers show non-random X-inactivation in B cells due to selection against the active mutant X during haematopoiesis.
● *clinical features* – a combined defect in cellular and humoral immunity presents in infancy with recurrent infections resistant to therapy. Bone marrow transplantation has been attempted by prognosis is poor.

X-linked hypogammaglobulinaemia
● *incidence* – rare.
● *genetic pathology* – caused by mutations in the BTK gene (Xq).
● *clinical features* – a B cell deficiency causing susceptibility to bacterial infections. Treatment involves infusion of human gammaglobulin.

Inborn error of metabolism

Ornithine transcarbamylase deficiency
● *incidence* – 1 in 70 000.
● *genetic pathology* – caused by mutations in the OTC gene (Xp).
● *clinical features* – deficiency of a critical enzyme in the urea cycle results in high blood ammonia levels, coma and early death in boys.

Intellectual handicap

Fragile X syndrome
See Chapter 8, Case 8.1.

Neurological malformations

X-linked hydrocephalus
● *incidence* – rare.
● *genetic pathology* – caused by mutations in the L1CAM gene (Xq).
● *clinical features* – severe hydrocephalus with aqueduct stenosis, agenesis of the lateral corticospinal tracts, adducted thumbs and mental retardation.

Neuromuscular disorders

Duchenne muscular dystrophy
See Chapter 7, Case 7.2.

X-LINKED DOMINANT DISORDERS

Oro-facio-digital syndrome
● *incidence* – rare.
● *genetic pathology* – unknown.
● *clinical features* – usually presents at birth with intraoral clefts, aberrant hyperplastic oral frenula and digital malformation (e.g. syndactyly or clinodactyly). Mental retardation may be a feature. This disorder is interesting because almost all affected cases are female with the sex ratio in unaffected sibs being 2:1 (f:m). It is though that males with this disorder cannot complete development and are miscarried.

Y-LINKED DISORDERS

Hypertrichosis of the ear rims (hairy ears)
- *incidence* – unknown.
- *genetic pathology* – unknown.
- *clinical features* – the Y-linked nature of hairy ears remains controversial. In a true Y-linked disorder there is only male to male transmission and all the sons of an affected man would be affected.

MITOCHONDRIAL DNA DISORDERS

MERRF
- *incidence* – rare.
- *genetic pathology* – caused by mutations in the mitochondrial genome (see Chapter 8, Box 8.2). ~80% of MERRF is caused by A to G mutation in the tRNA(leu) gene at nucleotide 8344.
- *clinical features* – *m*yoclonic *e*pilepsy associated with *r*agged *r*ed *f*ibers (MERRF); age and severity of dis-

ease presentation can vary greatly within families.

MELAS
- *incidence* – rare.
- *genetic pathology* – caused by mutations in the mitochondrial genome (see Chapter 8, Box 8.2). Approximately 80% of MELAS is caused by A to G transition at nucleotide 3243 in the tRNA-leu gene.
- *clinical features* – *m*itochondrial *m*yopathy, *e*ncephalopathy, *l*actic *a*cidosis and *s*troke-like episodes (MELAS). Symptoms include vomiting, seizures, and neurological insults resembling strokes.

Leber's hereditary optic neuropathy
See Chapter 8, Case 8.3.

CHROMOSOMAL DISORDERS

See Chapter 2, Boxes 2.3 and 2.4

Answers

ANSWERS to Chapter 1

1 *In the family tree shown in Fig. 1.7*
a **True.**
b **False.**
c **True.**
d **False.**
e **False.** *Sex unknown.*

2 *In the family tree shown in Fig. 1.8*
a **False.** *There is male to male transmission.*
b **True.** *She has an affected father and an affected son.*
c **True.**
d **True.** *It is unusual for an autosomal dominant disease to affect one sex more severely than the other (so called sex-limited). This family has more male members than female and chance is a more likely explanation for the observed inheritance pattern.*
e **True.**

3 *In the family tree shown in Fig. 1.9*
a **True.**
b **False.** *One in four or 25%.*
c **False.** *III-3 is unaffected so there is a 2 in 3 or 67% chance of being a carrier.*
d **True.**
e **True.**

4 *In the family tree shown in Fig. 1.10*
a **True.** *They are first cousins.*
b **False.** *They are monozygotic twins.*
c **False.** *Consanguinity is associated with an increased risk of recessive disorders.*
d **True.**
e **True.**

ANSWERS to Chapter 2

1 *Human chromosomes*
a **False.** *Chromosomes are complex structures of DNA, proteins, polyamines and metals.*
b **False.** *The number of chromosomes in each nucleus show considerable differences between species, e.g. muntjac deer have only six chromosomes in each cell, mice have 40 and rhinoceri 84.*

Humans happen to have 46.
c **False.** *Chromosomes are confined to the nucleus of the cell except during mitosis.*
d **False.** *Chromosomes are present in all nucleated cells.*
e **True.** *Giemsa- or G-banding allows the identification of individual chromosomes.*

2 *Human chromosome analysis by light microscopy*
a **False.** *Chromosome analysis can be performed on almost any dividing cells and is commonly done on skin fibroblasts, amniocytes and chorionic villus cells.*
b **False.** *Conventional analysis is not possible when chromosomes are decondensed and is usually done with the cells blocked in metaphase.*
c **False.** *Although some forms of computer analyses are currently possible, clinical cytogeneticists analyse all clinical samples 'manually'.*
d **True.** *The resolution of high-quality chromosome analysis by light microscopy is ~4×10^6 base-pairs.*
e **True.** *In ~5% of couples with three or more early miscarriages one partner will carry a chromosomal translocation.*

3 *Trisomy of chromosome*
a **False.** *Trisomy 21 is usually the result of an error in maternal first meiotic division.*
b **False.** *There is no association with increased paternal age in autosomal trisomies although there is a clear maternal age effect.*
c **False.** *The three human trisomies compatible with postnatal life, chromosomes 13, 18 and 21, all result in recognizable clinical phenotypes associated with growth failure, congenital malformations and mental handicap.*
d **False.** *Trisomy 13 occurs in 1 in 3000 births.*
e **False.** *Most pregnancies with trisomy 21 occur in women <30 years old. Although the risk of Down syndrome increases in women over 35 years of age the overall number of pregnancies in this group is considerably fewer than in younger women.*

4 *If the chromosomal constitution of an individual was*
a **False.** *In a 46,XX, normal female X-inactivation*

would have occurred in the preimplantation embryo and only one X chromosome is active in each cell.

b False. 45,X (Turner syndrome) have normal female external genitalia.

c True. All men with 47,XXY (Klinefelter syndrome) are infertile.

d False. Women with 47,XXX (Triple X syndrome) have normal fertility.

e True. Significant short stature is a very common feature of Turner syndrome.

5 Reciprocal translocations

a False. Reciprocal translocations can occur between any chromosomes.

b False. Reciprocal translocations are usually inherited.

c True. Translocation-associated disease is rare in carriers, although this may occur if a critical gene is interrupted by one of the breakpoints.

d True. In most cases there is a significant reproductive risk of chromosome aneuploidy in offspring of carriers.

e True. Male infertility in carriers is thought to result from a block in meiosis caused by formation of complex chromosomal pairing structures.

6 FISH analysis

a True. Interphase analysis on uncultured cells is likely to be a common application for FISH analysis in the future.

b True. A UV-light source with filters allowing excitation and visualization of fluorochromes must be attached to the microscopes.

c True. This is one of the most common clinical uses of FISH analysis to detect microdeletions in genomic DNA ($<1 \times 10^6$).

d False. FISH analysis is currently used as a second-line investigation in most cases after light microscopy. Newer FISH techniques which allow colour-coding of each chromosome pair may make this a first-line investigation in the future.

e True. One of the main research uses of FISH is to chromosomally localize (map) genes.

7 Robertsonian translocations

a True. rob(13;14) accounts for ~75% of all Robertsonian translocations.

b False. They involve fusion of the short arms of acrocentric chromosomes.

c True. It is not clear why there is a higher reproductive risk in female carriers than male carriers of Robertsonian translocations.

d False. Robertsonian translocations are rare (<5%

of cases) but important causes of trisomy 21 and 13.

e True. Dicentric chromosomes are a common feature of Robertsonian translocations.

8 Extra structurally abnormal chromosomes (ESAC)

a False. ESACs containing euchromatic material usually result in a clinical phenotype.

b True. Approximately 50% of all ESACs contain chromosome 15 material.

c True. Chromosome painting (**Box 2.17**) can be used to identify the chromosomal origin of the ESAC genetic material.

d True. iso(22q) can cause cat-eye syndrome.

e False. ESACs may be inherited through several generations.

9 Down syndrome

a True. Presenile dementia is a common problem in older people with Down syndrome.

b False. Down syndrome shows very little differences in incidence between races making environmental factors in the aetiology unlikely.

c True. Atrioventricular septal defects is one of the most common malformations in Down syndrome.

d False. Causes a predisposition to leukaemia.

e False. The Down syndrome critical region is on 21q22.2.

10 Giemsa–pale bands (R-bands) on human metaphase chromosomes

a True. Almost all the widely expressed human genes map to euchromatic regions.

b True. R-bands are GC-rich (~60% of the bases are either guanine or cytosine in these regions), whereas Giemsa-dark bands (G-bands) tend to be AT-rich.

c False. Constitutive heterochromatin (C-bands) contain tandemly repeated segments of DNA.

d False. C-bands are commonly involved in heteromorphisms, benign R-band variants are very rare.

e False. The X chromosome contains R-bands and G-bands like all normal human chromosomes.

ANSWERS to Chapter 3

1 Which of the following are features of the structure of human DNA?

a True.

b True. Both are double-stranded and made from the same sugar and bases. However, bacteria and mammals modify their DNA after synthesis in different ways. In mammals, methylation of cytosine at the sites of CG dinucleotides is the main form of modification. Also, mammalian and bacterial DNA are topologically different in that a bacterial 'chromosome' is a large closed circle of ds DNA, while mammalian chromosomes are linear.

c **False.** The deoxyribose sugars, not the bases, are connected by phosphates (see Fig. 3.1).

d **False.** A pairs with T (thymine). U (uracil) is present in RNA in place of T.

e **True.** 'Antiparallel'.

2 The following are consequences of the double-stranded structure of DNA

a **True.** The strands are complementary.

b **False.** Only some sequences will be palindromes (meaning that the sequence on both strands is the same).

c **True.**

d **True.** But usually in a given region of DNA only one of the two strands is the coding strand.

e **False.** Some are transcribed from one and some from the other strand. Genes transcribed from opposite strands also, of course, point in opposite directions along the length of the chromosome.

3 The following are true of restriction endonucleases

a **False.** They are isolated from microorganisms, mostly bacteria but also a few algae.

b **False.** Some restriction enzymes share a recognition sequence; they are termed isoschizomers. This is true, for example, of BspDI and ClaI, which both cut the sequence ATCGAT.

c **True.**

d **True.** Several restriction enzymes can tolerate alternative bases at one or more positions in their recognition sequence. For example, HincII cuts any site matching the sequence GT(C or T)(A or G)AC.

e **True.** Many restriction enzymes will not cut if one or more specific residues within the recognition sequence is methylated. For example, HpaII and MspI both recognize the sequence CCGG, but HpaII will not cut if the C of the central CG dinucleotide is methylated.

4 DNA and chromosomes

a **False.** The DNA within a human chromosome is a linear dsDNA molecule.

b **True.** This is collectively known as satellite DNA. One type of repetitive DNA known as **alphoid** satellite consists of tandem repeats of a 171 bp

unit, and is an important structural component of the centromere.

c **True.** There are two chromosomal homologues, each with two sister chromatids – four copies of each gene in all. (Exceptions to this would include most of the X chromosome in male cells, and those genes such as ribosomal RNA genes, which are present at more than one copy per haploid genome.)

d **False.** It is sister chromatids which separate from each other.

e **False.** Though most is, there is a small circular dsDNA genome within the mitochondria (see Chapter 8).

5 The polymerase chain reaction

a **True.** The thermal cycling procedure requires a DNA polymerase which can be added at the start of the reaction, resist the 95 °C denaturation step, and perform DNA synthesis at 72 °C. The most widely used such polymerase (Taq polymerase) was first isolated from the thermophilic bacterium Thermus aquaticus.

b **True.**

c **True.** By careful optimization, as little as one molecule of starting target DNA can yield a result. This fact is starting to be exploited to allow preimplantation genetic diagnosis, in which one cell of an in vitro fertilized embryo is removed and tested for a specific genetic abnormality.

d **True.** PCR can work with tiny quantities of poor quality DNA, such as may be obtained from the scene of a crime.

e **True.** If the RNA is first copied or 'reverse transcribed' into cDNA, then PCR can be performed. This is usually known as RT-PCR, and is a useful tool for examining the expression of a chosen gene.

6 Mutations

a **True.** Though this is unusual. See discussion of achondroplasia in Case 3.2.

b **True.** Allelic heterogeneity.

c **True.** For example Duchenne muscular dystrophy (deletion detectable in about 70%, remainder point mutations).

d **False.** A cause for the occurrence of a new mutation is rarely apparent.

e **False.** If the mutation being sought has been previously defined, simpler tests such as analysis of a restriction enzyme site altered by the presence of the mutation may be applicable.

7 Splicing

a **False.** These are the first and last two bases of an intron.

b **True. Alternative splicing** is a process whereby different patterns of exons within a gene may be spliced together. Some exons may be selected for splicing into mRNA as mutually exclusive alternatives, or some mRNAs may be made by simply omitting or skipping one or more exons. As a result, various non-identical proteins can be generated from a single gene.

c **False.** Most do, but a few do not.

d **False.** In the nucleus before mRNA export.

e **False.** Not all exons consist of a multiple of three nucleotides. Consequently not all encode an exact number of amino acids.

8 Genes

a **True.**

b **True.** Evolution progresses partly through duplication of ancestral genes followed by divergence of the sequences of the duplicated copies. Many genes can be grouped by sequence similarity into families of related structure.

c **True.** Some genes encode a functional RNA, e.g. transfer RNA, ribosomal RNA.

d **False.** The main structural features of some proteins have been maintained since the early days of evolution. Consequently, for some enzymes and the genes which encode them, it is possible to align the homologous human and bacterial sequences and demonstrate their common evolutionary origin.

e **False.** There is no known upper limit, and some have many more (>50).

ANSWERS to Chapter 4

1 If a disease displays allelic heterogeneity

a **False.** May be the only practicable way of analysing a family.

b **False.** Can still be useful if one or more mutations is known to be common or if resources are available to screen for unknown mutations.

c **False.** Means that several different mutations within the same gene can cause the disease.

d **False.** Many patients with autosomal recessive diseases have two different mutations in their two allelic copies of the disease gene. (They are then referred to as compound heterozygotes.)

e **True.** Though precise genotype–phenotype correlations are not always possible.

2 DNA polymorphisms

a **True.** Many thousands of polymorphisms on every chromosome.

b **True.** Are the landmarks used to construct genetic (as opposed to physical) maps, in which the genome is laid out according to the recombination frequencies between neighbouring landmarks.

c **False.** Detection of the mutation causing the disease must be used to confirm a doubtful diagnosis.

d **False.** Loss or gain of a restriction site is only one way of typing some polymorphisms (especially single base changes). Most VNTR polymorphisms are typed by PCR without use of restriction enzymes.

e **False.** Are a part of the individual's genetic constitution, and the same in all cell types.

3 Variable number tandem repeat polymorphisms (VNTRs)

a **True.** The larger number of possible alleles makes heterozygosity more likely.

b **False.** Are very common, and are the most widely used tool in diagnostic molecular genetics (especially CA repeats).

c **True.** 'Slippage' during DNA replication results in occasional alteration in repeat number between generations. For CA repeats, mutation rates are between 0.001 to 0.01 per generation.

d **True.** Presence of several VNTR alleles in a child which are absent from a putative father and from the mother is the usual way of disproving paternity.

e **True.** Heterozygosity is the proportion of individuals who have distinguishable alleles for a given polymorphism. Heterozygosity >90% implies an extremely informative polymorphism. The CA repeat polymorphisms used for most human genetic work have heterozygosities in the range of 65–90%.

4 Polymorphisms

a **False.** They also occur in exons, including coding regions, where they may or (more often) may not alter the amino acid sequence of the encoded protein. However, the lack of selective pressure against most sequence changes in introns means that polymorphisms are more common in introns than exons.

b **False.** Amino acid sequence variants occur in many proteins. They may or may not alter the biochemical properties of the protein discernibly.

c **False.** The polymorphism will be transmitted with the standard Mendelian probability of 0.5. The son will also have a probability of 0.1 of inheriting the same variant from his mother. His overall chance of inheriting the variant from one or both parents *will be 0.55.*

d **True.** *Visible variation in size is particularly common in the heterochromatic regions near the centromeres of some chromosomes such as 9, and in the short arms of the acrocentric chromosomes. It may allow the parental origin of the chromosomal homologues to be distinguished.*

e **True.** *Chromosome 21 polymorphisms may indicate from which parent the extra 21 originated, and also at which meiotic division the error occurred.*

5 Crossing over

a **False.** *Only if diagnosis by linkage to a polymorphic marker is being used.*

b **False.** *It is not the informativeness but the genetic distance from the mutation which matters.*

c **False.** *Occurs in both. However, recombination frequencies between any two markers are not the same in male and female meiosis.*

d **False.** *In female meiosis, may involve any part of the X, and in male meiosis, occurs between X and Y in the small pseudoautosomal region at the tip of the short arm.*

e **False.** *Sites of recombination are variable, giving rise to probabilities of recombination between two markers which are related to their distance apart.*

6 The following are true of diagnosis by use of linked markers

a **True.**

b **True.** *Though not in all cases, this is often necessary.*

c **True.** *Though there may still be a finite risk of crossing over within the gene, between the mutation site (unknown) and the site of the polymorphism.*

d **True.**

e **False.** *Allelic heterogeneity is not a problem; locus heterogeneity is.*

7 The following diseases are known to display locus heterogeneity

a **True.**

b **True.**

c **False.**

d **False.**

e **False.**

ANSWERS to Chapter 5

1 Neonatal screening for biochemical genetic disorders

a **False.** *Neonatal screening is best done after*

establishment of normal feeding, usually ~6 days of life.

b **False.** *Screening for PKU became widely available in the UK in the early 1960s.*

c **False.** *Neonatal screening is most often performed on dried blood or capillary samples from a heel-prick blood test.*

d **False.** *Results of the screening must be available within a few days as diseases such as PKU or congenital hypothyroidism require prompt treatment to avoid handicap.*

e **False.** *Most neonatal screening programmes are organized at a regional or national level using centralized testing facilities to ensure consistency of results.*

2 Huntington's disease is

a **True.** *Caudate atrophy is a consistent neuropathological finding in Huntington's disease and can be seen on MRI scans during life.*

b **False.** *HD is rarely diagnosed in childhood, ~5% of cases present before the age of 20 years.*

c **True.** *Psychiatric symptoms can be one of the most debilitating features of HD.*

d **False.** *HD has a mean age of onset of 35 years.*

e **True.** *See Case 5.4.*

3 Adult polycystic kidney disease (APKD)

a **True.** *APKD causes symptoms in ~50% of gene carriers.*

b **False.** *APKD has an incidence of 1 in 1000 births.*

c **True.** *Mutations in the polycystin gene on 16p and an unknown gene on chromosome 4 cause APKD.*

d **True.** *Berry aneurysm formation is relatively common.*

e **True.** *Approximately 10% of patient on dialysis programmes have APKD.*

4 Acute intermittent porphyria (AIP)

a **False.** *AIP is an autosomal dominant disorder.*

b **True.** *May be triggered by many environmental factors incuding infections, alcohol and drugs which upregulate ALA synthetase.*

c **False.** *Is caused by deficiency of porphobilinogen deaminase.*

d **False.** *Is an extremely rare cause of acute psychosis as AIP has an incidence of ~1 in 50 000.*

e **True.** *Increased levels of δ-aminolevulinic acid (ALA) and porphobilinogen (PBG) can be found on urine testing during acute attacks.*

5 Drug-induced decompensation is a feature of the following disorders

a True. Malignant hyperpyrexia can be triggered by specific anaesthetic agents, alcohol, exercise and infection.

b True. Glucose-6-phosphate dehydrogenase deficiency may be triggered by many different drugs including primaquine.

c False. Tay–Sachs disease has no specific drug sensitivities.

d False. C1 esterase inhibitor deficiency is the cause of angioneurotic oedema which is not usually drug-induced.

e True. Butyrylcholinesterase deficiency is the cause of suxamethonium sensitivity.

6 Phenylketonuria

a False. Causes accumulation of phenylalanine in the plasma and a relative deficiency of tyrosine.

b False. The biochemical severity does not specifically improve with age but is dependent on the genetic defect and the dietary therapy.

c False. Most cases are picked up by the national screening programme and treatment should start before 2 weeks of age.

d False. The offspring of a mother with untreated PKU commonly have microcephaly and heart defects.

e True. A relative deficiency of tyrosine is thought to cause a pigmentary disorder resulting in fair hair and blue eyes.

7 Presymptomatic testing in genetic diseases by DNA analysis

a False. Should be performed where there is a demand from at-risk relatives.

b False. PST can be done in relatives of affected individuals at any risk.

c False. PST may be done in children if there is a medical advantage to the child of an early diagnosis.

d True.

e True. PST is possible in familial cancer syndromes where the underlying defect is known or linkage is possible.

8 Phenotypic testing in genetic diseases

a True. Can prevent morbidity by leading to early treatment, e.g. hypertension in APKD.

b False. For APKD phenotypic screening is best done by abdominal ultrasound.

c False. Uses physical features rather than genetic analysis.

d True. In familial cancer syndromes such as familial adenomatous polyposis coli phenotypic screening may be performed using colonoscopy for polyp formation or ophthalmoscopy for hypertrophy of the retinal pigment epithilium.

e False. It is usually difficult to definitively exclude carrier status using phenotypic screening.

ANSWERS to Chapter 6

1 Amniocentesis

a True. CVS is more prone to placentally derived artifacts.

b False. There is no increased risk of a chromosome abnormality.

c False. Amniocentesis is performed trans-abdominally.

d True. Depending on the operator's experience.

e True.

2 Ultrasound scanning

a True. Although other neural tube defects are rarely apparent before 16 weeks.

b False. There is no firm connection between ultrasound and any fetal malformation.

c True. Although it is rarely possible to diagnose the type.

d True.

e True.

3 Chorionic villus sampling is the investigation of choice for women with

a False. Small familial translocations can be missed on CVS. Amniocentesis is more reliable.

b True.

c False. Ultrasound and/or amniocentesis should be considered to look for neural tube defects and anterior abdominal wall defects.

d True.

e True.

4 A raised maternal serum AFP is associated with the following fetal malformations

a True.

b False. Low maternal serum AFP is common in Down syndrome pregnancies.

c True.

d True.

e False.

ANSWERS to Chapter 7

1 In an X-linked recessive disease

a False. They may be new mutations.

b **False.** There is a 50% risk of such a daughter being a carrier.

c **False.** There is no risk of the son inheriting a mutation from his father. However, he still has the general population risk of being affected, as a result of a new mutation or maternally inherited mutation.

d **False.** The proportion of cases which are new mutations is different for each individual disorder. This proportion actually depends on the reproductive fitness of affected individuals and on the ratio of the mutation rates in male vs. female gametogenesis. Though the proportion varies, for all X-linked recessive diseases, inherited cases outnumber new mutations.

e **True.** This is really the definition of recessive for an X-linked disease. It is, however, theoretically possible for a female to be affected if homozygous for a mutation; this is a highly unlikely scenario given the low frequency of X-linked mutations in the population. Occasional apparently affected females may result if there is extreme skewing of the ratio of X-inactivation, or as a result of X-autosome translocations which allow only the structurally normal X to be inactivated.

2 The following are true of haemophilia

a **True.** In haemophilia A, in addition to the common inversion mutation described above, there are many point mutations described, and some deletions. In haemophilia B too, there is a wide range of mutations, mostly point mutations.

b **True.** Haemophilia A (F8C) and haemophilia B (F9C).

c **False.** Bisects the gene and therefore causes severe disease.

d **False.** The mutation usually occurs during spermatogenesis and therefore appears de novo in girls but not usually boys. These carrier girls can then transmit the mutation to have affected sons.

e **True.** Possibly the first example of genetic linkage reported in man, by J.B.S. Haldane. Both F8C and RGCP, the genes cluster encoding the red and green opsin pigment proteins, which are deficient in colour blindness, lie in Xq28.

3 The following are true of Duchenne muscular dystrophy

a **True.** This derives from another result obtained by Haldane. He showed that for a lethal X-linked disease, the loss of mutations from the population must be balanced by a steady supply of new mutations (or the disease would die out). If the male and female mutation rates are approximately equal (as for DMD but not haemophilia), it can be calculated that one-third of isolated cases will result from such new mutations.

b **True.** In Becker dystrophy, onset is later and progress of the disease slower. Somewhat surprisingly, many Becker patients have large deletions of the dystrophin gene. There is evidence that the difference between Becker deletions and those in Duchenne patients is that in the former the exons which are missing are such as to allow the remaining exons of the gene to be spliced together without disturbing the amino acid reading frame (i.e. an exact multiple of 3 bp is removed). This allows synthesis of a shortened but still partially functioning protein. In Duchenne dystrophy the deletions are out of frame and result in virtual absence of functional protein.

c **True.**

d **True.** Provided that a deletion is the cause of the disease within that family, then FISH with a probe located within the deletion will allow detection of a deleted X chromosome by absence of FISH signal.

e **True.** The dystrophin gene is huge (2.2 million bp). The recombination fraction between polymorphisms located at opposite ends of the gene is approximately 0.12 (12 cM). Even when using intragenic markers for linkage, appreciable error rates have to be considered.

4 The following are true of X inactivation

a **True.** The inactive X becomes heavily methylated in association with its transcriptional silencing. It is detection of methylation which allows assessment of the pattern of X inactivation in the laboratory.

b **True.** Equal status has to be restored to the two X chromosomes prior to meiosis, so that either can be transmitted in a functional state to the ovum.

c **False.** Spreads from an inactivation centre on Xq. The pseudoautosomal region is at the tip of Xp.

d **True.** Occurs in any cell with more than one X chromosome.

e **False.**

5 Which of the following may result in apparent skewing of the pattern of X inactivation?

a **True.** A significant proportion of unselected normal women show skewing of X inactivation in favour of one X by a ratio 10 : 90 or greater when peripheral blood DNA is examined.

b True. As for carriers of X-SCID in lymphocytes. Presumed to be because the gene product in question is needed for cell survival.

c True. Since inactivation spreads from an inactivation centre to involve the rest of the chromosome, if this happened on a translocation chromosome it would result in functional monosomy for the translocated autosomal segment. Since this would be lethal, there is strong selection in favour of inactivating the normal (untranslocated) X.

d False.

e False. Though may be observed by chance.

ANSWERS to Chapter 8

1 Which of these statements applies to Fragile X syndrome?

a False. The expanded CGG repeat is outside the coding region of the FMR1 protein. Rather than an abnormal protein being produced therefore (as in Huntington's disease), the effect of triplet expansion is to shut down transcription. Affected boys therefore have a deficient amount of FMR1 protein.

b False. Only by DNA testing.

c False. Normal transmitting males pass their premutations to their daughters, who are therefore all carriers of premutations, but unaffected. Expansion to full mutation only occurs on maternal transmission.

d True. Because of post-zygotic instability of the full mutation (in the early embryo), many affected boys are mosaics, with some cells carrying full and some pre-mutations.

e True. There are rare cases of individuals in whom the deficiency of FMR1 results not from triplet expansion but from a point mutation within the gene. This proves that it is loss of FMR1 function, and not some additional effect, which causes Fragile X syndrome.

2 The following are true of mitochondria and mitochondrial inheritance

a False. Only a few are. Many proteins made in the cytoplasm from nucleus-derived mRNAs are imported into the mitochondrion after synthesis.

b True.

c True. This reflects the evolutionary origin of mitochondria as ancient bacteria 'captured' by the eukaryotic cell. Some codons have different functions from their nuclear equivalents e.g. UGA ('stop' codon in nuclear mRNAs) encodes trypto-

phan in mammalian mitochondria.

d True. The mitochondrion usually performs oxidative metabolism of pyruvate derived from glycolysis. If oxidative metabolism is defective, then pyruvate is converted instead to lactate.

e True. See text.

3 Cryptic translocations

a True.

b True.

c True.

d False.

e False. An unbalanced translocation carrier, if fertile, may transmit the derivative chromosome he/she is carrying (producing unbalanced offspring).

4 Imprinted genes

a True. Though this may occur only in some tissues.

b False. There are a number of large imprinted 'domains' which contain several imprinted genes.

c False. Only a small number (100) genes are believed to be imprinted.

d False. The gene is normally inherited, in one copy from each parent. Its pattern of methylation and expression is determined by the parent of origin.

e True.

5 Uniparental disomy

a False. No phenotype is associated with UPD for some chromosomes.

b False. Only occasionally may the occurrence of unusual structural chromosome variants allow the demonstration of UPD by cytogenetics.

c True.

d True.

e False. Some human UPDs have never been reported. Some may result in early embryonic lethality, hence escaping detection.

6 Gonadal mosaicism

a True. A recognized problem in Duchenne muscular dystrophy. For example, a male who is an unaffected gonadal mosaic may transmit a mutation to several daughters.

b True. Its existence can usually only be suspected, but the possibility means that recurrence risks for mutations not present in either parent usually higher than the general population risk.

c True. Only occasionally done.

d False.

e True. Though in practice very difficult to prove.

ANSWERS to Chapter 9

I Familial cancer syndromes
a True. *Most cases result from a somatic mutation.*
b True. *Most are dominant (e.g. von Hippel Lindau) although a few are recessive (ataxia telangiectasia).*
c True. *Li Fraumeni syndrome which causes a variety of cancers including leukaemia and ovarian cancer is associated with germ-line p53 mutations.*
d True. *Although not invariably.*
e False. *Translocations are a common feature of sporadic haematological malignancies (Philadelphia chromosome).*

2 Breast cancer
a True.
b False. *vHL is characterized by central nervous system, retinal and renal tumours.*
c False. *Most cases are sporadic.*
d True.
e False. *Mammographic screening is offered to women over 50 as part of the National Breast Screening Programme.*

3 Mutations in
a True. *In HNPCC.*
b False. *Usually somatic.*
c True.
d True.
e True. *Somatic mutations in p53 have been implicated in the pathogenesis of lung cancer in smokers.*

4 Direct gene testing
a False. *Only possible in families in which a mutation has been identified.*
b True.
c False. *Requires the expertise of a Regional Molecular Genetic Centre.*
d True.
e True. *RNA tests are technically more complex and harder to reproduce accurately.*

5 Chromosome breakage syndromes
a True. *Some studies suggest that carriers of ataxia telangiectasia have an increased breast cancer risk.*
b True.
c True. *Fanconia anaemia may be associated with radial aplasia and other malformations.*
d False. *Usually recessive.*
e False. *Acute lymphatic leukaemia is the commonest childhood cancer.*

6 Knudson's two-hit hypothesis
a True.
b False. *Tumour suppressor gene action.*
c True.
d True.
e False. *Refers to the inactivation of tumour suppressor genes.*

ANSWERS to Chapter 10

I Syndrome diagnoses
a True. *The consistency of the patterns of abnormalities differentiates syndromes from associations.*
b True. *This large number of different conditions reflects the complexity of human development.*
c True. *Syndrome diagnoses are often eponymous, i.e. are named after an individual (e.g. Down syndrome, Edward's syndrome) usually the first person to report the disorder; several attempts have been made to replace the eponym as a naming device for syndromes, sequences and dysplasias but these have, so far, been unsuccessful.*
d False. *Developmental field defects involve local abnormalities in adjacent tissues of different embryological origins.*
e False. *Pathophysiology of most syndromes is unknown.*

2 The neural tube
a True.
b False. *The cause of most neural tube defects (NTD) is not known although a defect in folic acid metabolism is suspected.*
c False. *The neural tube begins to fuse in the middle with progression of fusion in both cranial and caudal directions.*
d True.
e True. *Sodium valproate result in NTD in ~1% of exposed pregnancies.*

3 Human teratogenic effects
a True. *Sodium valproate may cause NTD, digital anomalies and unusual facies.*
b False. *From ethanol are seen ~ 1 in 500 births.*
c False. *Vitamin A (retinoic acid) is a potent teratogen.*
d True. *Warfarin may result in nasal hypoplasia and chondrodysplasia punctata.*
e False. *Any teratogenic effect in the first 3 weeks after fertilization is thought to be lethal to the embryo. Organogenesis (4–8 weeks) is the most sensitive period for most teratogens.*

4 Monozygous twins

a False. Conjoined twins are extremely rare.

b False. MZ twins are genetically identical whereas double-first cousins share 25% of their genes.

c True. Comparisons of twin concordance between MZ and DZ twins can be used to calculate the genetic contribution to common disorders.

d False. MZ twins with an adult-onset genetic disease are unlikely to develop symptoms at exactly the same age, probably as a result of environmental factors influencing the phenotype.

e True. MZ twins have an increased risk of birth defects.

5 Limb development

a False. Is apparent by 26 days of gestation.

b True. Limb development can be interrupted by many teratogens. The most famous of these is thalidomide-induced phocomelia.

c True. Programmed cell death is necessary to produce separation of the digits in the developing hand and foot.

d False. Begins in the upper limb at 26 days and the lower limbs 2 days later.

e False. The ZPA on the opposite side to the thumb and appears to be an important control region for the normal patterning of the digits.

6 The developing kidney

a False. Is primarily derived from mesoderm.

b True. The mesonephric duct contributes to the male genital tract as the vas deferens and epididymis.

c False. Renal aplasia is the primary malformation in Potter's sequence with secondary deformations occurring in other systems.

d False. Is morphologically complete by 58 days of gestation.

e False – Is a relatively common site for human malformations.

7 Birth defects

a False. Occur in ~3 in 100 live births.

b False. Approximately ⅓ of cases are due to known chromosomal and single-gene defects.

c True. In most children birth defects involve only one organ system.

d True. Malformations are a common feature of chromosomal abnormalities.

e False. Malformations, deformations, disruptions and dysplasias are all birth defects.

8 Preimplantation period of development

a False. There is little overall growth of the preimplantation embryo.

b True. The inner cell mass forms in the blastocyst towards the end of the preimplantation period.

c False. Most malformations occur considerably later in development during organogenesis.

d False. Preimplantation lasts ~1 week.

e True. Preimplantation development can be partly accomplished in vitro and this is clinically useful in certain fertility treatments.

9 Computer programs to aid dysmorphic diagnoses

a True. One of the main advantages of computer use is the ability to perform complex searches using combinations of birth defects.

b True. Searching for specific diagnosis is best done with pivotal features which are often relatively unusual clinical findings, e.g. radial aplasia or polydactyly.

c False. Computers are not yet able to match facial photographs and this remains one of the main skills in dysmorphology.

d True. It is now impossible for any individual to retain all the clinical details of all possible dysmorphic diagnoses and computer searches are particularly useful in matching features in very rare disorders.

e False. These computer programs are now an integral part of most dysmorphologists' clinical practice.

10 The diagnostic features of

a False. A sequence is a single-site defect that results in apparently unrelated defects (e.g Potter's sequence, Case 10.2) and a developmental field complex has features that are restricted to a single anatomical site (e.g. hemifacial microsomia).

b True. Dysplasic processes are likely to be progressive (e.g. skin abnormalities in mucopolysaccharidoses).

c False. A syndrome may have a purely behavioural phenotype (e.g. Smith–Magenis syndrome).

d False. Hemifacial microsomia is a developmental field complex involving defects tissues derived from several germ layers.

e True. Many syndromes show considerable phenotypic overlap, e.g. Noonan syndrome was described as male Turner syndrome due to the neck webbing and short stature seen in both conditions.

Index

Page numbers in *italic* refer to illustrations and tables; **bold** page numbers indicate a main discussion.